First Edition

CELLULAR ENGINEERING

A Laboratory Manual

Sakthikumar Ambady

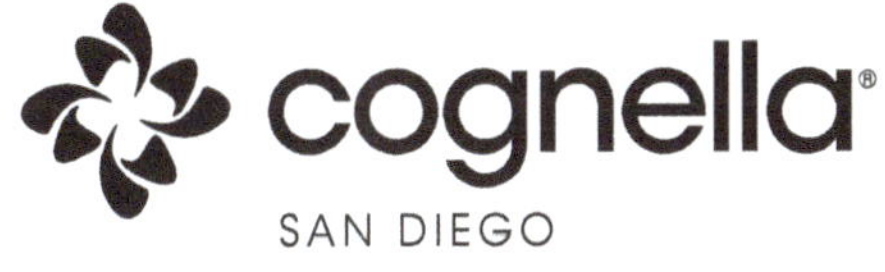

Bassim Hamadeh, CEO and Publisher
John Remington, Executive Editor
Gem Rabanera, Senior Project Editor
Jeanine Rees, Production Editor
Emely Villavicencio, Senior Graphic Designer
JoHannah McDonald, Licensing Coordinator
Natalie Piccotti, Director of Marketing
Kassie Graves, Senior Vice President, Editorial
Alia Bales, Director, Project Editorial and Production

Printed in the United States of America.

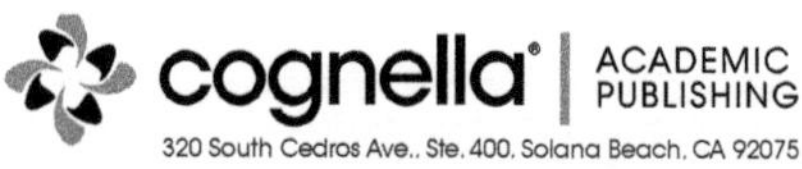

Brief Contents

Detailed Contents

UNIT I

The Basics

Chapter 1

The History of Cell Culture

CHAPTER PURPOSE

This chapter introduces students to some of the landmark events that were instrumental in bringing cell culture to the forefront of research in life sciences, medicine, biotechnology, and allied fields.

CHAPTER APPLICATION

Students will develop an appreciation of the advancements and improvements that have occurred in the field of cell culture in the last few decades. Students are encouraged to refer to the original literature to gain a deeper understanding of the efforts that have gone into bringing cell culture and cellular engineering to its current prominence.

From the Humble Beginnings of Cell Culture to 3D Bioprinting of Tissues and Organs

Cell culture has become an indispensable tool for research in life sciences, medicine, biotechnology, and other allied fields. From the humble beginnings from the laboratory of Ross Granville Harrison at Yale University in 1907, where he described the culture of frog nerve cells, animal cell culture has come a long way. Primary cells and cell lines derived from normal and diseased tissues are helping scientists understand basic biology, develop cell therapies for various diseases, and manufacture biologics for medical and industrial applications. The development of mouse-induced pluripotent stem cells (iPSCs) in 2006 and human iPSCs in 2007 heralded a new era in stem cell research and regenerative medicine. The discovery of the ability of CRISPR-Cas9 complex to effect precise manipulation of genes promises to revolutionize our ability to correct gene defects in cells both in vitro and in vivo.

The earliest record of in vitro animal cell culture dates to the report presented by Ross Granville Harrison at the Proceedings of the Society for Experimental Biology and Medicine in 1907 and published as a journal publication in 1910 (Harrison, R. G. (1907); Harrison, R. G (1910)). He described the culture of frog nerve cells in a fibrin clot using a technique called the "hanging drop" method. In this method, he attached tissue fragments to glass coverslips and covered it with partially coagulated serum or lymph. The coverslips were placed upside down in a humidified chamber to produce the hanging drop. This technique allowed the direct observation of cells under a microscope. However, the hanging drop method did not permit long-term cultures under aseptic conditions. In 1911, Alexis Carrel started cell culture from connective tissue of blood vessels, heart, skin, muscles, peritoneum, and spleen of 14-to-20-day-old chick embryos. He wanted to "determine the conditions under which the active life of a tissue outside of the organism could be prolonged indefinitely." He hypothesized that "senility and death of the cultures, instead of being necessary, resulted merely from preventable occurrences, such as accumulation of catabolic substances and exhaustion of the medium." In his opinion, it was possible to extend the life of cultured cells in vitro because "elemental death might be postponed indefinitely by a proper artificial nutrition." The culture medium he used composed of Ringer's solution and hypotonic plasma. He initially performed cultures in two "phases" : (a) a proliferative phase at 38 °C, during which the cells used up the medium, proliferated, and were surrounded by catabolic products; (b) a latent phase at 0 °C, during which the cells remained idle and culture medium could be exchanged. In later experiments, the latent phase was avoided so that the life of the tissues was continuous and the growth more rapid. The final technique he employed involved placing a 1-cm^2 piece of silk veil on a cover glass moistened with a drop of plasma. A small piece of tissue was placed on the silk veil and covered with a few drops of plasma. The hollow side was sealed and cultured in an incubator. After a few days, a piece of tissue, along with the piece of silk, was "transplanted" to new vessels with fresh plasma. Up to 20 "transplantations" were conducted for each culture (Carrell, 1912). He describes the behavior of the culture as follows:

> [T]he fragment of tissue was surrounded rapidly by cells spreading in a thin layer through the medium. After section of the plasma, the new tissue retracted around the original fragment, forming an opaque crown. During the period of washing, there was no modification of the culture, but as soon as the culture was put in a new medium in the incubator, elongated cells began to grow from the edges of the old plasma and to spread into the new medium. After a few passages, the original fragment appeared diminished in size and surrounded by a dense envelope of a greyish tissue from which radiated a great many elongated cells, living and dead.

In 1922, Albert Ebeling, an associate of Carrel, who took charge of Carrel's cultures in 1912, reported 10 years of continuous culture of chick embryo heart cells from January 17, 1912, to January 17, 1922 (Ebeling, 1922). He reported the existence of 60 cultures that represented the 1,860th generation of the original cells. Ebeling continued the cultures and was able to maintain the cells in continuous culture for 34 years. They were finally terminated in 1946. Apart from developing the cell culture method, Carrel pioneered the development of glass tissue culture flasks that had a flat bottom, a rounded body, and an oblique neck that was easy to sterilize using the Bunsen burner. He needed a system wherein "tissues and fluids are easily introduced with a pipette, and particles of dust cannot fall into the culture medium while the flask is opened" (Carrel, 1923).

Carrel's training as surgeon prepared him to follow aseptic techniques in his cell culture work. One criticism of Carrel's work was that others were unable to replicate his "immortalized" chick embryo culture. It has been hypothesized that fresh cells were inadvertently added to Carrel's cultures every time fresh plasma was added to replenish the medium. The growth and proliferation of these freshly added cells kept the cultures going, leading to the impression that the cells were immortal. This notion continued until Hayflick and Moorhead (1961) proposed the cellular senescence theory of primary cells (known as the "Hayflick limit"). It was not until the 1990s that the scientific community accepted Hayflick's findings that primary cells have a limited lifespan (Hayflick, 1998).

Modern-day cell culturists owe a great deal of gratitude to the pioneering works of researchers and scientists who developed the procedures to isolate and expand cells in vitro, develop cell lines, and formulate cell culture media to meet specific nutritional requirements for specific cell types. Some of the pioneering works include those of Earle et al. (1943; mouse L-cells), Gey et al. (1952; HeLa cells), Puck et al. (1958; CHO cells), and Todaro and Green, (1963; NIH/3T3 cells), to name a few. Most of these initial cell cultures were started using homemade culture media. For example, HeLa cells were cultured in a composite medium of chicken plasma, bovine embryo extract, and human placental cord serum. CHO cells were cultured in a mixture of 40% N16 medium, 15% fetal calf serum, 1% antibiotic solution containing a mixture of penicillin, streptomycin, and tertramycin, 4% NCTC 109 solution and saline F solution (a mixture of glucose and balanced salt solution) to make up the rest of the volume. By 1963, Todaro and Green reported using Dulbecco's modification of Eagle's medium (DMEM) supplemented with 10% calf serum. The early cell line development was followed by the development of mouse embryonic stem cells in 1981 and human embryonic stem cells in 1998. The ethical dilemma of using ES cells produced from developing embryos was mitigated after the development of human induced pluripotent stem cells (iPSCs) in 2006 (mouse) and 2007 (human). This paved the way for the development of organoids and embryoids in vitro. Organoids and embryoids can be generated from adult, embryonic, and induced-pluripotent stem cells, and they reflect the physiological and genetic properties of the cell type(s) they are derived from. Embryoid bodies aid in the study of embryonic development and modeling mammalian development from preimplantation stage of embryos to early organogenesis. Organoids exhibit structural, morphogenetic, and functional properties that resemble those of their in vivo counterparts. This is helping scientists understand the normal physiology of cells and changes associated with genetic defects.

Tissue and organ engineering have garnered much attention in recent years. Biomedical engineers are using iPSCs to repopulate decellularized organs. 3D printing of tissues and organs using a combination of natural and synthetic biomaterials in conjunction with a variety of 3D printing technologies is being pursued for organ engineering. The technology has not yet achieved the kind of print resolution required to print and create functional tissues and organs. The ability to print capillary beds at the desired resolution remains the biggest challenge to 3D bioprinting. It will require expertise from biologists, chemists, biochemists, material scientists, and varied engineering fields to realize the full potential of 3D bioprinting. The future is promising, and the road to success is paved with many challenges. Table 1.1 lists some of the landmark discoveries and inventions that has brought cell culture technology to where it is today.

TABLE 1.1 Major Milestones in Cell Culture, Media Development, and Biomedical Technologies

Year	Event
1665	Robert Hooke publishes *Micrographia* and uses the term "cell" for the first time.
1676	Antoni van Leeuwenhoek presents the results of his microscopic observations in a letter to the Royal Society.
1830s	Botanist Matthias Schleiden and zoologist Theodor Schwann formulate the "cell theory."
1855	Rudolph Virchov states the theory of tissue formation "Omnis cellula-e-cellula," or "All cells come from cells."
1907	Ross Granville Harrison establishes the hanging drop culture method for frog embryo nerve fibers in vitro.
1910	Alexis Carrel, and Montrose Burrows cultured explants of tissue fragments for 2–3 months.
1912	Alexis Carrel establishes aseptic techniques for cell cultures.
1912–1946	Alexis Carrel and Albert H. Ebeling conducted long-term culture of chick heart tissue cells
1916	Peyton Rous and F.S. Jones use trypsin to subculture cells.
1920	The European Collection of Authenticated Cell Culture (ECACC) is established.
1925	The American Type Culture Collection (ATCC) is established.
1930s	Alexis Carrel develops new cell culture devices.
1943	The first continuous fibroblast cell line, L-cells, is established from mouse connective tissue.
1943	Wilton Robinson Earle and coworkers develop a balanced salt solution that forms the base for several culture media.
1948–1952	Keilova-Rodova (1948) and Cruickshank and Lowbury (1952) report the use of antibiotics in tissue culture.
1948	Katherine K. Sanford, Wilton R. Earle, and Gwendolyn D. Likely derive clone L929 from a mouse L-cell line.
1950	J. F. Morgan develops Medium 199 to cultivate chicken embryonic cells under protein-free conditions.
1952	George O. Gey, Ward D. Coffman, and Mary T. Kubicek report the establishment of HeLa cell line, derived from a cervical carcinoma cancer patient, Henrietta Lacks.
1955	Harry Eagle formulates the "defined" cell culture medium called "Basal Medium Eagle" (BME) for mouse L-cells and human HeLa cells.
1957	Theodore T. Puck and colleagues report the development of Chinese hamster ovary (CHO) cells.
1957	CMRL 1066 media is developed by modifying Medium 199 to culture mouse L-cells under protein-free conditions.
1957	The National Cancer Institute develops the NCTC109 medium for culturing mouse L-cells under protein-free conditions.
1958	Stewart H. Madin and Norman B. Darby, Jr develop the Madin-Darby canine kidney (MDCK) cell line.
1959	Harry Eagle publishes the composition of "minimal essential medium" (MEM).

Year	Event
1959	Renato Dulbecco and G. Freeman report the development of "Dulbecco's modified minimal essential medium" (DMEM).
1959	Thomas McCoy develops McCoy's 5A Modified Medium to culture Novikoff hepatoma cells.
1959	Waymouth's MB 752/1 medium was developed to grow cells in a serum-free environment.
1961	Leonard Hayflick and Paul S. Moorhead propose the finite lifespan of cells (Hayflick limit).
1962	Ian Macpherson and Michael Stoker report the development of BHK-21 cells from a Syrian hamster kidney.
1962	George Todaro and Howard Green report the development of NIH/3T3 cells.
1962	Yasumura, Y and Kawakita, Y report the development of Vero cell line from the kidney of an African green monkey.
1963	Richard G. Ham develops Ham's F-10 media to enable colony formation by a single Chinese hamster ovary (CHO) cell under serum-free conditions.
1963	Leibovitz's L-15 medium is formulated to maintain pH at an ambient environment outside a CO_2 incubator.
1964	Ham's F-12 medium is developed, credited as the world's first chemically defined medium.
1965	Henry Harris and J.F. Watkins report the viral fusion of human and mouse cells, a precursor to hybridoma technology.
1966	The Roswell Park Memorial Institute media (RPMI 1640) is developed, a modification of McCoy's 5A Medium, for the long-term culture of peripheral blood lymphocytes.
1964	Glen Fischer reports the development of Fischer's Medium for the culture of mouse leukemic cells.
1970	J.P. Jacobs, C.M. Jones, and J.P. Baille report their study on MRC-5 cells from human lungs.
1971	Development of a-MEM media, modified for use for hybrid-cell-line research.
1973	J.L. Biedler, L. Helson and B.A. Spengler report the development of SK-N-SH cells from the bone marrow biopsy of a 4-year-old female with neuroblastoma (precursor to subclone SHSY-5Y cell line).
1973	H.D. Soule. J. Vazguez, A. Long, S. Albert, and M. Brennan report the development of MCF-7 breast cancer cell line from the pleural effusion of a 69-year-old woman with metastatic breast cancer.
1973 to 1977	Development of human embryonic kidney 293 cell line (HEK293) in Alex van der Eb's laboratory.
1974	Kaighn's modified Ham's F-12 (Ham's F-12K) medium is developed.
1975	Georges J.F. Köhler and César Milstein report the development of hybridoma cell lines.
1976	Lloyd Greene and Arthur S. Tischler report the development of PC12 cells from pheochromocytoma of the rat adrenal medulla.
1976–1984	Several versions of molecular, cellular, and developmental biology (MCDB) media were formulated that were optimized for the growth and proliferation of specific cell types.

Year	Event
1978	N.N. Iscove reports the development of "Iscove's modified DMEM" (IMDM) media, suitable for high-density cultures and cultures of rapidly proliferating cells.
1978	David Goeddel and his colleagues at Genentech produce recombinant human insulin from the combination of A and B chains individually expressed in E. coli.
1978	J.L. Biedler, S. Roffler-Tarlov, M. Schachner, and L.S. Freedman report the derivation of a SHSY-5Y subclone from SK-N-SH cells.
1978	R. Cailleau, R. Young, M. Olivé, and W.J. Reeves Jr. report the establishment of MDA-MB-231 breast cancer cell line from a 51-year-old Caucasian female with a metastatic mammary adenocarcinoma.
1979	DMEM/F-12 medium is developed, a 50:50 mixture of Ham's F-12 and DMEM media for use as a basal medium for serum-free culture.
1981	M.J. Evans and M.H. Kaufman report the development of mouse ES cells.
1981	Yakov Gluzman develops COS cells (CV-1 [simian] in origin and carrying the SV40 genetic material). Three lines—COS-1, COS-3 and COS-7—were generated.
1982	Michael W. McBurney and Brenda J. Rogers report the development of P19 mouse embryonal carcinoma cells.
1984	RPMI 1640/DMEM/F-12 (RDF) media for the serum-free culture of hybridomas is developed. It is a mixture of RPMI 1640, DMEM, and Ham's F-12 at a ratio of 2:1:1.
1987	Michele Calos's lab at Stanford University publishes their work on HEK293T cells, established by the expression of a temperature-sensitive SV40 T-antigen mutant.
1987	The first human recombinant therapeutic protein—tissue plasminogen activator (r-tPA, Activase)—is produced in CHO cells for clinical use.
1993	Kjell Bertheussen reports the use of protein-free media for cell culture.
1998	James Thomson's group reports the isolation of human embryonic stem cells from IVF embryos.
2005	Jinyou Zhang and David Robinson report the use of animal-free, protein-free, and chemically defined media for antibody production.
2006	Kazutoshi Takahashi and Shinya Yamanaka report the development of mouse iPSCs.
2007	James Thomson's group reports the development of human iPSCs.
2008	Mototsugu Eiraku and colleagues report the development of 3D cerebral cortex tissue organoid from embryonic stem cells.
2008–present	Various organoids are developed using mouse and human ES cells and iPSCs. For reviews, see Corrò et al. (2020), Tang et al. (2022), Zhao et al. (2022), and Calà et al (2023).
2010	The first "organ-on-a-chip" lung model is reported by Donald Ingber from Harvard's Wyss Institute.
2010	Anthony Atala's group demonstrates 3D tissue and organ bioprinting.
Since 2010	3D bioprinting is in various stages of development using different printing technologies.

References

Calà, G., Sina, B., De Coppi, P., Giovanni, G. G., & Gerli, M. F. M. (2023). Primary human organoids models: Current progress and key milestones. *Frontiers in Bioengineering and Biotechnology, 11*. https://doi.org/10.3389/fbioe.2023.1058970

Carrel, A. (1912). On the permanent life of tissues outside of the organism. *Journal of Experimental Medicine, 15*(5), 516–28. https://www.doi.org/10.1084/jem.15.5.516. PMID: 19867545; PMCID: PMC2124948.

Carrel, A. (1923). A method for the physiological study of tissues in vitro. *Journal of Experimental Medicine, 38*(4), 407–18. https://www.doi.org/10.1084/jem.38.4.407. PMID: 19868798; PMCID: PMC2128453.

Corrò, C., Novellasdemunt, L, & Li, V. S. W. (2020). A brief history of organoids. *American Journal of Physiology Cell Physiology, 319*(1), C151–C165. https://www.doi.org/10.1152/ajpcell.00120.2020. PMID: 32459504; PMCID: PMC7468890.

Dey, M., & Ozbolat I. T. (2020). 3D bioprinting of cells, tissues and organs. *Scientific Reports, 10*(1), 14023. https://www.doi.org/10.1038/s41598-020-70086-y. PMID: 32811864; PMCID: PMC7434768.

Ebeling, A. H. (1922). A ten year old strain of fibroblasts. *Journal of Experimental Medicine., 35*(6), 755–59. https://www.doi.org/10.1084/jem.35.6.755

Earle, W. R., Schilling, E. L., Stark, T. H., Straus, N. R., Brown, M. F., & Shelton, E. (1943). Production of malignancy in vitro: The mouse fibroblast cultures and changes seen in the living cells. *Journal of the National Cancer Institute, 4*, 165–212.

Gey, G. O., Coffman, W. D., Kubicek M. T. (1952). Tissue culture studies of the proliferative capacity of cervical carcinoma and normal epithelium. *Cancer Research, 12*, 264–65.

Gillmore, J. D., Gane, E., Taubel, J., Kao, J., Fontana, M., Maitland, M. L., Seitzer. J., O'Connell, D., Walsh, K. R., Wood, K., Phillips, J., Xu, Y., Amaral, A., Boyd, A. P., Cehelsky, J. E., McKee, M. D., Schiermeier, A., Harari, O., Murphy, A., Kyratsous, C. A., ... Lebwohl, D. (2021). CRISPR-Cas9 in vivo gene editing for transthyretin amyloidosis. *The New England Journal of Medicine, 385*(6), 493–502. https://www.doi.org/10.1056/NEJMoa2107454. PMID: 34215024.

Harrison, R. G. (1907). Observations on the living developing nerve fiber. *Proceedings of the Society for Experimental Biology and Medicine, 4*, 140–43.

Harrison, R. G. (1910). The outgrowth of the nerve fiber as a mode of protoplasmic movement. *Journal of Experimental Zoology, 9*, 787–846.

Hayflick, L., Moorhead, P. S. (1961). The serial cultivation of human diploid cell strains. *Experimental Cell Research*, 585–621. https://www.doi.org/10.1016/0014-4827(61)90192-6. PMID: 13905658.

Hayflick, L. (1997). Mortality and immortality at the cellular level. A review. *Biochemistry (Mosc), 62*(11), 1180–90. PMID: 9467840.

Hayflick, L. (1998). A brief history of the mortality and immortality of cultured cells. *The Keio Journal of Medicine, 47*(3), 174–82. https://www.doi.org/10.2302/kjm.47.174. PMID: 9785764.

Jedrzejczak-Silicka, M. (2017). History of Cell Culture. In S. J. T. Gowder (2017), *New Insights Into Cell Culture Technology*. https://www.doi.org/10.5772/66905

Puck T. T., Cieciura S. J., & Robinson A. (1958). Genetics of somatic mammalian cells III: Long-term cultivation of euploid cells from human and animal subjects. *Journal of Experimental Medicine, 108*(6), 945–56. https://www.doi.org/10.1084/jem.108.6.945. PMID: 13598821; PMCID: PMC2136918.

Takahashi, K., & Yamanaka, S. (2006). Induction of pluripotent stem cells from mouse embryonic and adult fibroblast cultures by defined factors. *Cell, 126*(4), 663–76. https://www.doi.org/10.1016/j.cell.2006.07.024. PMID: 16904174.

Tang, X. Y., Wu, S., Wang, D., Chu, C., Hong, Y., Tao, M., Hu, H., Xu, M., Guo, X., & Liu, Y. (2022). Human organoids in basic research and clinical applications. *Signal Transduction and Targeted Therapy, 7*(1), 168. https://www.doi.org/10.1038/s41392-022-01024-9. PMID: 35610212; PMCID: PMC9127490.

Todaro, G. J., & Green, H. (1963). Quantitative studies of the growth of mouse embryo cells in culture and their development into established lines. *Journal of Cell Biology, 17*(2), 299–313. https://www.doi.org/10.1083/jcb.17.2.299. PMID: 13985244; PMCID: PMC2106200.

Zhao, Z., Chen, X., Dowbaj, A. M,, Sljukic A, Bratlie K, Lin L, Fong ELS, Balachander GM, Chen Z, Soragni A, Huch M, Zeng YA, Wang Q, Yu H. (2022). Organoids. *Nature Reviews Methods Primers*, 2(94). https://doi.org/10.1038/s43586-022-00174-y

■ Chapter 2

Cell Culture Basics

CHAPTER PURPOSE

This chapter provides an overview of the basic equipments and the safety precautions for a biosafety-level-1 (BSL-1) lab.

CHAPTER APPLICATION

"Cell culture" refers to the process of maintaining cells derived from a variety of sources in an environment that closely mimics the requirements for the specific cell type. This chapter describes the basic equipments used in cell culture labs and informs the students about the need to take safety precautions while dealing with live cells of human and animal origin.

Lab Safety Guidelines

Any individual working with biological materials must adhere to the principles of biosafety introduced in 1984 by the Biosafety in Microbiological and Biomedical Laboratories (BMBL) and the safety regulations prescribed by individual institutions. The guidelines address the safe handling and containment of infectious microorganisms and hazardous biological materials. Their guidance is based on the occurrence of laboratory-associated infections (LAI) evidenced through a series of research publications between 1951 and 1978 (Sulkin & Pike, 1951; Pike et al.,1965; Pike, 1976, 1978). These studies reported that the 10 most common causative agents of overt infections among workers handling biological materials were *Brucella* species, *Coxiella burnetii*, hepatitis B virus (HBV), *Salmonella enterica* serotype *Typhi*, *Francisella tularensis*, *Mycobacterium tuberculosis*, *Blastomyces dermatitidis*, Venezuelan equine encephalitis virus, *Chlamydia psittaci*, and *Coccidioides immitis*. These findings support the notion that cell cultures have the potential to cause health risks to research personnel. Based on these findings, the Centers for Disease Control (CDC) formulated the concept of biosafety levels (BSL) 1 to 4. Infographics of the four biosafety levels and detailed procedures are presented in Appendix I and II respectively. In general, teaching labs are designated either as BSL-1 (infectious agents or toxins not known to consistently cause disease in healthy adults) or BSL-2 (moderate-risk infectious agents or toxins that pose a risk if accidentally inhaled, swallowed, or exposed to the skin). It is recommended that students working in a cell culture lab wear gloves, a lab coat, and safety goggles or other personal protective equipments (PPE) as prescribed by the safety office at the institution.

Equipment For a Cell Culture Lab

Biosafety Cabinets

The *biosafety cabinet* (BSC), otherwise called a laminar flow hood, is an essential part of the cell culture lab. BSCs serve three main purposes (a) protecting the personnel from potential pathogens harbored by the cells (b) protecting the cells from the personnel handling the cells and (c) protecting the cells from potential contaminants in the culture environment. For cell culture work, three classes of flow hoods are considered: class-I, class-II, and class-III BSCs. They provide various levels of safety protection to the personnel, specimen, and environment. General cell culture work involves dealing with specimens with biosafety levels 1, 2, and 3. In instances where protection should be provided to the personnel, specimen, and environment for student labs and most research labs, class-II BSCs are used (Table 2.1). Diagrammatic representation of airflow in a class-II, type-A BSC used in student cell culture labs is presented in Figure 2.1. Specifications of the different classes of BSCs, such as face velocity, airflow pattern, and recommendations on the use of volatile and nonvolatile chemicals and radionuclides, are presented in Table 2.2.

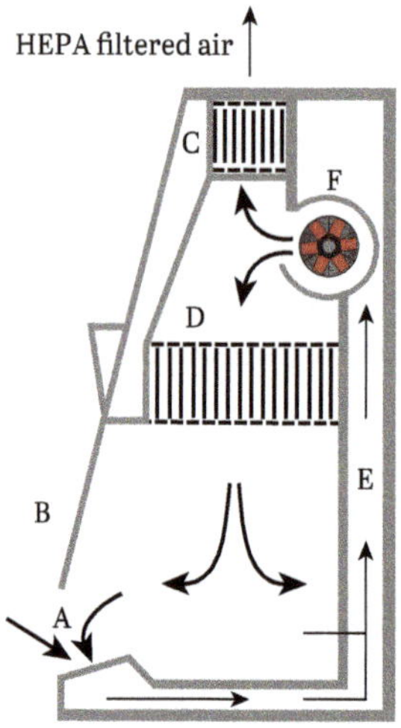

FIGURE 2.1 The Class-II, Type-A Biosafety Cabinet: (a) Front Opening; (b) Sash; (c) Exhaust HEPA Filter; (d) Supply HEPA Filter; (e) Common Plenum; and (f) Exhaust Blower. Ambient air is taken through the front grill, filtered through the HEPA filter, and distributed to the cabinet. The flow pattern produces an air curtain at the front opening.

TABLE 2.1 Selection of a Safety Cabinet Through Risk Assessment

Biological risk assessed	Protection provided			
	Personnel	Product	Environmental	BSC class
BSL 1–3	Yes	No	Yes	I
BSL 1–3	Yes	Yes	Yes	II (A1, A2, B1, B2)
BSL 4	Yes	Yes	Yes	III; II - When used in suit room with suit

Source: Matthew J. Arduino et al., "Selection of a Safety Cabinet Through Risk Assessment," Biosafety in Microbiological and Biomedical Laboratories, *p. 388, 2020.*

TABLE 2.2 Comparison of Biosafety Cabinet Characteristics

BSC class	Face velocity (linear feet per minute, LFM)	Airflow pattern	Applications	
			Nonvolatile toxic chemicals and radionuclides	Volatile toxic chemicals and radionuclides
I	75	In at front through HEPA to the outside or into the room through HEPA	Yes	When exhausted outdoors[a, b]
II, A1	75	70% recirculated to the cabinet work area through HEPA; 30% balance can be exhausted through HEPA back into the room or to outside through a canopy unit[c]	Yes (small amounts)[b]	Yes (small amounts)[a, b]
II, A2	100	Similar to II, A1 but has 100 LFM intake air velocity and plenums are under negative pressure to room; exhaust air can be ducted to the outside through a canopy unit	Yes	When exhausted outdoors (formally "B3") (small amounts)[a, b]
II, B1	100	30% recirculated, 70% exhausted; exhaust cabinet air must pass through a dedicated, internal cabinet duct to the outside through a HEPA filter	Yes	Yes (small amounts)[a, b]
II, B2	100	No recirculation; total exhaust to the outside through a HEPA filter	Yes	Yes (small amounts)[a, b]
II, C1	100	30% recirculated, 70% exhausted; exhaust cabinet air must pass through a dedicated, internal cabinet duct to the outside through a blower and HEPA filter	Yes	Yes (small amounts)[a, b]
III	N/A	Supply air is HEPA filtered; exhaust air passes through two HEPA filters in series and is exhausted to the outside via a hard connection	Yes	Yes (small amounts)[a, b]

Source: Matthew J. Arduino et al., "Comparison of Biosafety Cabinet Characteristics," Biosafety in Microbiological and Biomedical Laboratories, p. 388, 2020.

[a]Installation requires a special duct to the outside and may require an in-line charcoal filter and/or a spark-proof (explosion-proof) motor and other electrical components in the cabinet. Discharge of a class-I or class-II, type A2 cabinet into a room should not occur if volatile chemicals are used.

[b]A risk assessment should be completed by laboratory and safety facility personnel to determine amounts to be used. In all cases, only the smallest amounts of the chemical(s) required for the work to be performed should be used in the BSC. In no instance should the chemical concentration approach the lower explosion limits of the compounds.

Cell Culture Incubators

Cell culture incubators are designed to provide a controlled environment for growing cells where parameters such as temperature (4 °C to 50 °C), humidity (95% to 100%), oxygen (ambient oxygen), and carbon dioxide (5–10%) levels can be maintained. Most research labs grow cells under ambient oxygen levels (~21%). Researchers studying the effect of hypoxia or hyperoxia use special incubators capable of controlling oxygen levels. The interior of the cell culture incubator is sealed by a heated glass door to prevent CO_2 and humidity leaks. The heated door prevents water condensation allowing visualization of the interior of the chamber (Figure 2.2). Air circulation inside the incubator is facilitated by a fan and helps distribute heat uniformly inside the chamber. Some of the specifications of cell culture incubators are presented in Table 2.3.

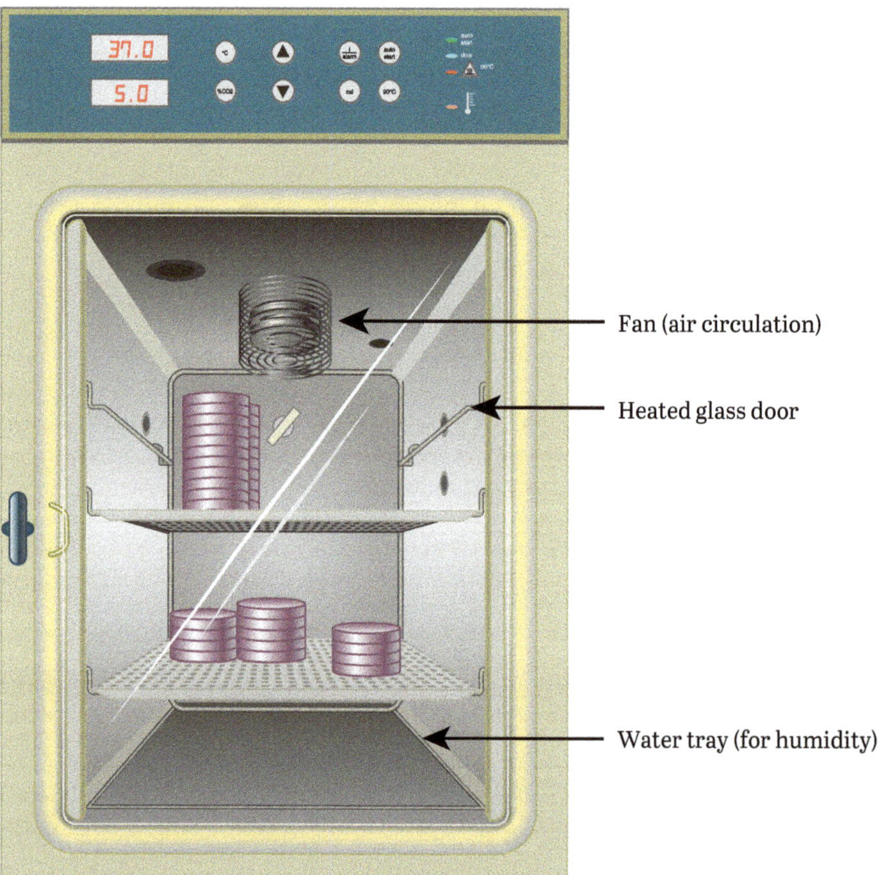

FIGURE 2.2 Air-Jacketed Cell Culture Incubator: (a) The Panel on the Incubator Displaying Temperature (37 °C) and CO_2 level (5%); (b) the Interior of the Incubator

TABLE 2.3 Incubator Sizes, Parameters, and Control Mechanisms

Feature	Model, system, or control
Incubator size	Benchtop model (1.5 to 6 cu ft)
	Floor model (5.5 to 9 cu ft)
	Large capacity Reach-in model (up to 29 cu ft)
Temperature control	Water jacketed
	Air jacketed
	Direct heat
Humidity control	Atomizer system
	Water reservoir
Decontamination	High heat
	UV light
	Hydrogen peroxide
Routine contamination control	Copper shelving
Carbon dioxide control	Infrared sensors
Oxygen control	Ambient air for regular cultures
	By varying levels of nitrogen in hypoxic incubators

Centrifuges

Centrifugation is a mechanical process in which a centrifugal force is applied to separate fluids of different densities or particles suspended in a solution. For the latter, the efficiency of separation depends on the size, shape, density, viscosity of the medium in which the particles are suspended, centrifugal force, mass, angular velocity, and the radius of rotation. In the context of cell culture, a centrifugation technique called "pelleting" is used to isolate cells from a cell suspension. Other centrifugation techniques used for various other applications include isopycnic centrifugation, ultrafiltration, density gradient, phase separation, and continuous flow centrifugation.

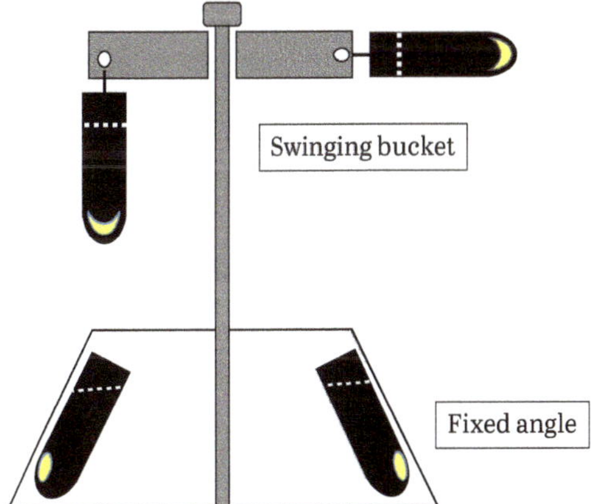

FIGURE 2.3 Types of Centrifuges: Swinging Bucket and Fixed-Angle Rotor. Notice the differences in the pelleting behavior between the two types of centrifuges.

A centrifuge is composed of a chamber that houses the rotor and the electric motor. Tube holders are attached to the rotor assembly. The rotational force generated by the electric motor is transferred to the rotor and, subsequently, to the sample being centrifuged. The two most commonly used rotors in cell culture labs are (a) fixed angle rotors and (b) swinging bucket rotors (Figure 2.3). Cells will pellet differently depending on what type of rotor is used. Cells sediment at the bottom of the tube if a swinging bucket centrifuge is used.

In the fixed angle rotor centrifuge, cells sediment at the farthest point from the center. In fixed-angle rotor centrifuges, the tube should be oriented in such a way to make it easy to locate the cell pellet, particularly if fewer cells are used.

RPM vs. RCF

Revolutions per minute (RPM) represents the speed of the centrifuge rotor. RPM does not define the force exerted by the rotational force on the cells. *Relative centrifugal force* (RCF or g-force), on the other hand, represents the "force" exerted on the sample. In other words, RPM is a function of the speed of the rotor without considering the radius of the rotor. Therefore, the same RPM exerts a larger gravitational force on cells in a centrifuge with large radius compared to a centrifuge with smaller radius. RCF, on the other hand, is a universal value across all centrifuges regardless of the radius (Table 2.4). Most protocols and publications indicate RPM when describing the centrifugation method. Unless the radius of the centrifuge is known, it is impossible to calculate the "force" of centrifugation. If the radius is known, RCF can be calculated from RPM values using the following formula:

$$\mathbf{RCF = (RPM)^2 \times 1.118 \times 10^{-5} \times \mathit{r}}$$

Here, r is the maximum radius, expressed in centimeters.

From the above formula, it is evident that two centrifuges with different radius of rotation will exert vastly different g-forces for the same RPM value. Table 2.4 demonstrates this relationship, where two rotors of 6-cm and 10-cm radius are used. Higher g-forces can affect cell viability. Care should be taken to centrifuge the cells between 200 g and 250 g.

TABLE 2.4 The Relationship Between RPM and RCF

A different g-force is produced at the same RPM		
	Radius (6 cm)	Radius (10 cm)
RPM	14,000	14,000
RCF	**13,148 g**	**21,913 g**

A different RPM is produced at the same g-force		
	Radius (6 cm)	Radius (10 cm)
RCF	200 g	200 g
RPM	**1,727**	**1,338**

Note. Two centrifuges of different radius when set at the same RPM generate different g-forces (left Table). Conversely, to attain the same g-force, the RPM for the two centrifuges must be set differently (right Table).

Water Baths, Dry Baths, Incubators, and Heating Blocks

Water baths, dry baths, regular small incubators, or *dry heating blocks* maintained at 37 °C are used to warm up media, buffers, and other reagents used in cell cultures. Dry baths are preferred to water baths to avoid the risk of bacteriological contamination. If water baths are used, regular cleaning and disinfection are critical for preventing growth of contaminants in the water bath.

Hemocytometer

A *hemocytometer* is a device that was originally developed to count blood cells. Rapid advancements in the field of hematology in the 1800s were a major impetus in developing the hemocytometer. The device consists of a thick glass slide laser etched with 3 × 3 square grids of 1 mm^2 each and a raised edge with a height of 0.1 mm (Figure 2.4). The design of a blood cell counting device was first created by the German physician Karl Vierdordt in 1852, who described the use of a capillary tube to count cells. An improved method and a precursor to the modern hemocytometer was designed by the French anatomist Louis Charles Malassez in 1874. He described the use of flattened capillary tubes with rulings, glued to a glass slide. Further improvements were made by Ricard Thoma in 1881 and Karl Burker between 1905 and 1913. The most commonly used hemocytometer today is the Neubauer hemocytometer developed in 1907. Its configuration and the volumes of squares within the counting regions are presented in Figure 2.5. Recently, disposable hemocytometers (C-Chip) have become available. These are great alternatives to traditional hemocytometers due to their versatility and ease of use. Disposable hemocytometers are particularly useful in teaching labs. Automatic cell counters, if available, can be a great alternative to manual cell counting methods.

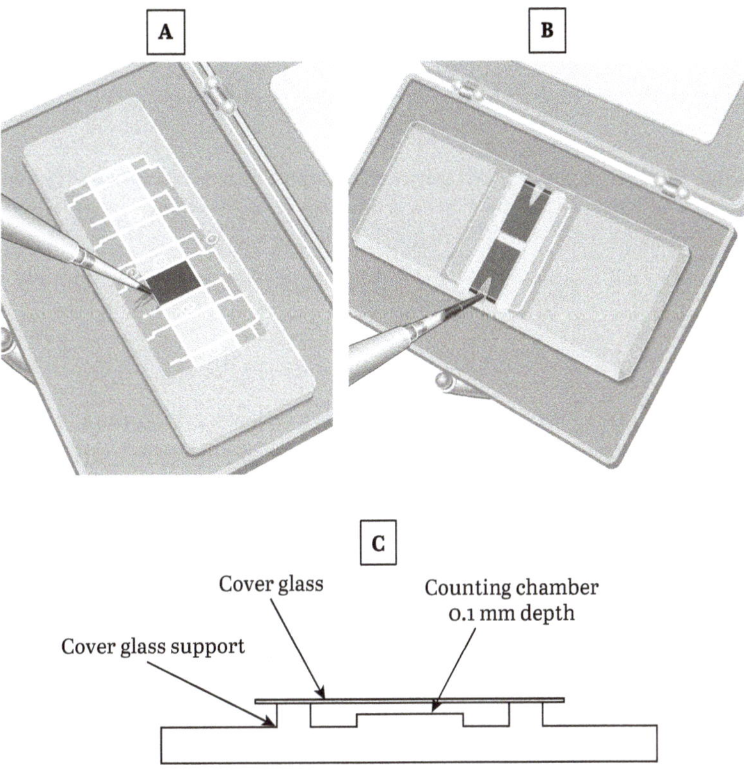

FIGURE 2.4 Hemocytometers: (a) C-Chip Disposable Hemocytometer With Four Counting Chambers, (b) Neubauer Hemocytometer; and (c) Diagrammatic Representation of the Neubauer Hemocytometer

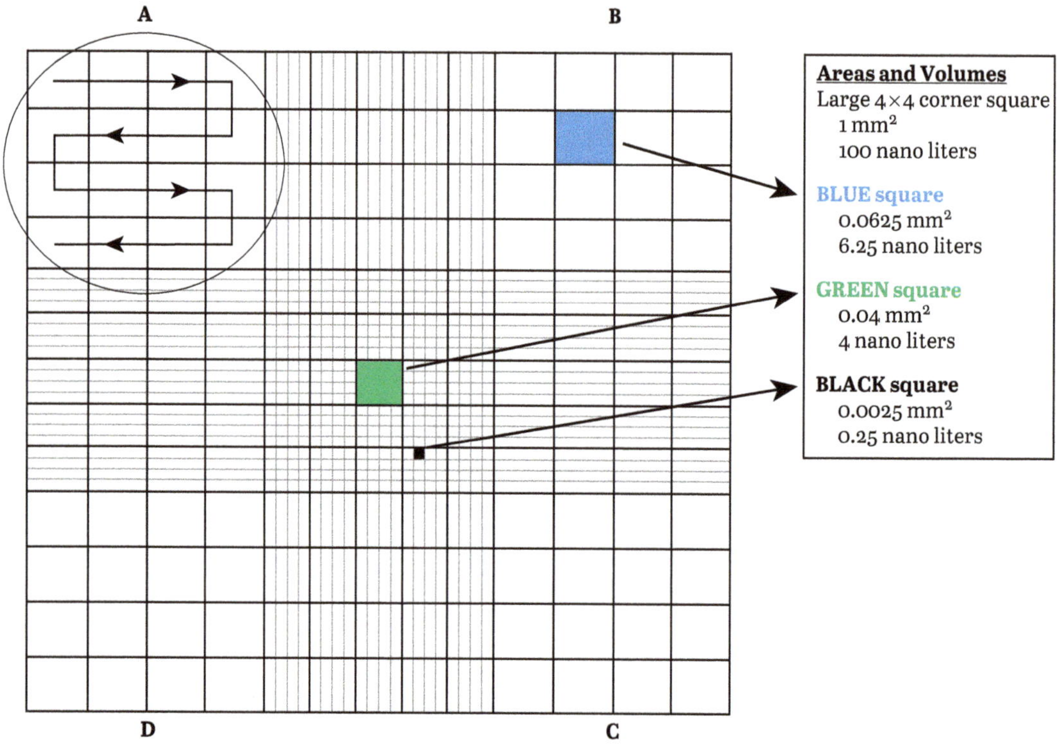

A
B
D
C

Areas and Volumes
Large 4×4 corner square
1 mm^2
100 nano liters
BLUE square
0.0625 mm^2
6.25 nano liters
GREEN square
0.04 mm^2
4 nano liters
BLACK square
0.0025 mm^2
0.25 nano liters

FIGURE 2.5 Grid Structure of Hemocytometers and Their Volumes. The corner squares A, B, C and D are used to count larger eukaryotic cells, such as fibroblasts. The center square is used to count smaller cells, such as red blood cells. Cell counting is done in a zigzag fashion, as depicted in corner square A. The volumes of corner squares and the smaller subdivisions within the larger squares are indicated.

Microscopes

A *microscope* is an essential component of any cell culture lab. Microscopes are used to check the quality of cells, cell proliferation, cell confluency and for detecting contamination. The most commonly used microscope for observing live cells is an inverted phase contrast microscope. Dutch physicist Frits Zernike won the Nobel prize in 1953 for his invention of phase contrast microscopy. His invention permitted the observation of live cells and their organelles, avoiding the need to fix the cells. Unstained specimens do not absorb light and are called "phase objects." When light passes through the specimen, a slight shift in their diffraction occurs that is imperceptible to the naked eye. The phase rings used in phase contrast microscopy are able to separate the illuminating light (background) from the specimen-scattered light to produce high contrast images. The main components of a phase contrast microscope are presented in Figure 2.6. The eye pieces provide 10 to 15-fold magnification. The commonly used objectives in phase contrast microscopes used for cell culture are 4x or 5x, 10x, 20x, and 40x objectives. Each objective has a collar that carries a universal color code to allow easy identification: red for 4x and 5x, yellow for 10x, green for 20x, and light blue for 40x (Figure 2.7). Phase contrast microscopes come with matching phase rings and objectives. To obtain the best images, the objectives should be used in conjunction with the correct phase ring (Figure 2.8).

Camera port
Light intensity switch
Coarse and fine focus
Microscope stage
Green filter
Condenser
Objectives
Phase rings
Eye pieces
On/Off switch

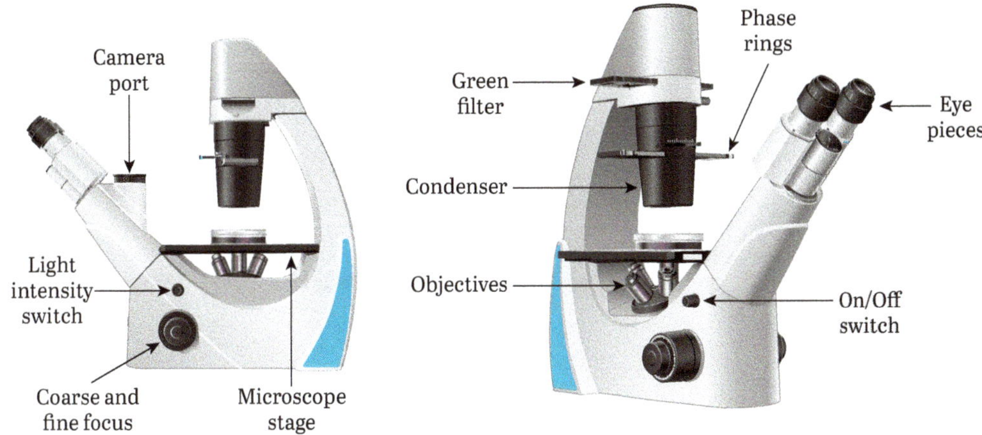

FIGURE 2.6 Inverted Phase Contrast Microscope and its Main Components

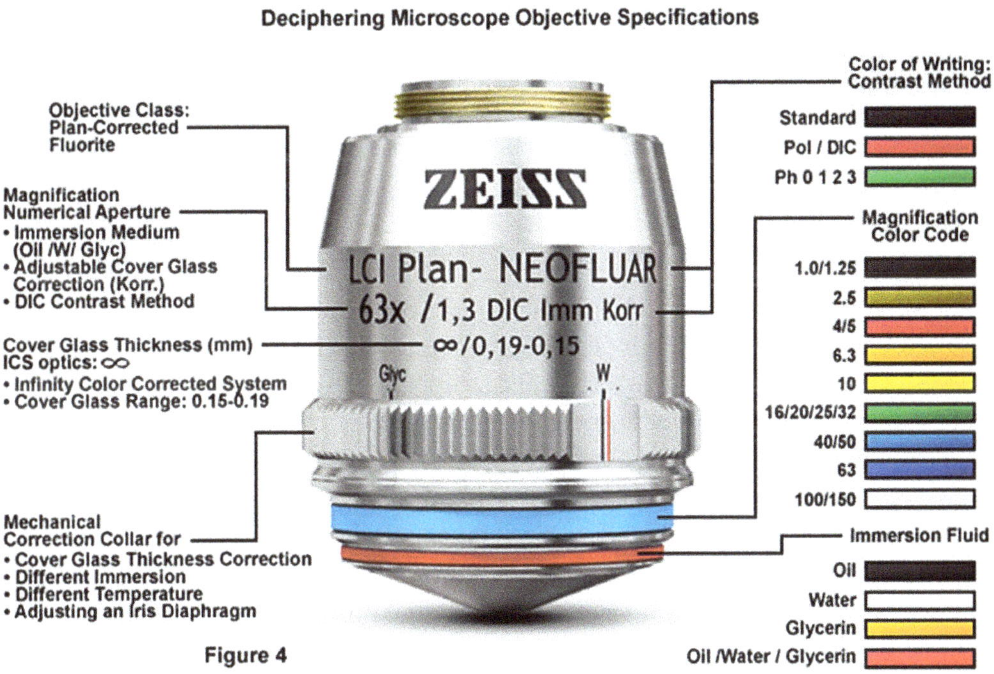

Deciphering Microscope Objective Specifications
Objective Class: Plan-Corrected Fluorite
Magnification Numerical Aperture
• Immersion Medium (Oil /W/ Glyc)
• Adjustable Cover Glass Correction (Korr.)
• DIC Contrast Method
Cover Glass Thickness (mm) ICS optics: ∞
• Infinity Color Corrected System
• Cover Glass Range: 0.15-0.19
Mechanical Correction Collar for
• Cover Glass Thickness Correction
• Different Immersion
• Different Temperature
• Adjusting an Iris Diaphragm
ZEISS
LCI Plan- NEOFLUAR
63x /1,3 DIC Imm Korr
∞/0,19-0,15
Glyc
W
Color of Writing: Contrast Method
Standard
Pol / DIC
Ph 0 1 2 3
Magnification Color Code
1.0/1.25
2.5
4/5
6.3
10
16/20/25/32
40/50
63
100/150
Immersion Fluid
Oil
Water
Glycerin
Oil /Water / Glycerin
Figure 4

FIGURE 2.7 Color Coding of the Objective Rings for Easy Identification of the Objective Magnification

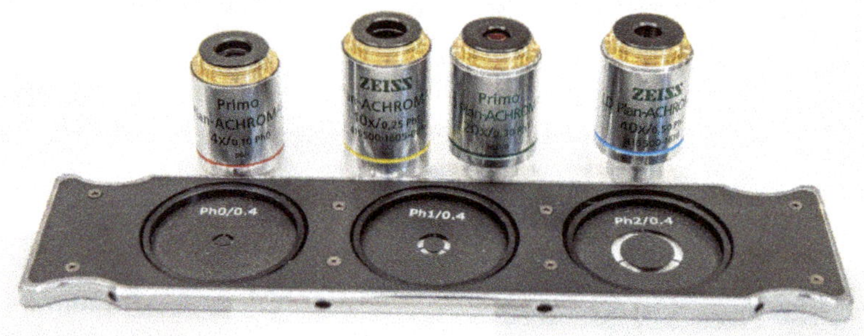

FIGURE 2.8 Phase Contrast Rings and Their corresponding Objectives for the Zeiss Primovert Microscope. The 4x and 5x objectives are used in conjunction with the left phase ring; the 10x and 20x objectives are used in conjunction with the middle phase ring; and the 40x objective is used in conjunction with the right phase ring.

Other Equipment

Other equipment for a cell culture lab include fridges, freezers, micropipettes, pipet aids, liquid nitrogen cell storage tanks, culture vessels, other consumables and personal protective equipments.

Chapter Takeaways

A good working knowledge of all lab equipments used for cell culture and the principles employed in the functioning of the equipment is key to success in a cell culture lab. For example, performance of water jacketed incubators versus air jacketed incubators; use of ambient oxygen versus hypoxic conditions; 5% CO_2 versus 10% CO_2 incubators; and temperature requirements for cells from various species. The type of biosafety cabinet used should correspond to the biosafety level of the type of specimen used in the lab. Understanding the proper use of microscopes is essential to obtaining good images. Understanding the use of imaging software is key to inserting scale bars and quantifying important parameters, such as cell size, cell morphology, nuclear–cytoplasmic ratio, and cell migration. Students must learn the importance of using RCF (g-force) instead of RPM as a standard practice to describe centrifugation speeds. RPM is equipment specific, whereas RCF is a universal measure. Students should adhere to institution-specific requirements regarding the use of personal protective equipment.

References

Centers for Disease Control and Prevention. (2020). *Biosafety in microbiological and biomedical laboratories* (6th ed.). https://www.cdc.gov/labs/BMBL.html

Pike, R. M., Sulkin, S. E., & Schulze, M. L. (1965). Continuing importance of laboratory-acquired infections. *American Journal of Public Health*, *55*, 190–99.

Pike, R. M. (1976). Laboratory-associated infections: Summary and analysis of 3921 cases. *Health Laboratory Science*, *13*, 105–14.

Pike, R. M. (1978). Past and present hazards of working with infectious agents. *Archives of Pathology & Laboratory Medicine*, *102*, 333–36.

Sulkin S. E., & Pike R. M. (1951). Survey of laboratory-acquired infections. *American Journal of Public Health*, *41*, 769–81.

Credits

Fig. 2.1: Matthew J. Arduino et al., "The Horizontal Laminar Flow Clean Bench," Biosafety in Microbiological and Biomedical Laboratories, 2020.

Fig. 2.4c: Ewen, "Hemocytometer Side," https://commons.wikimedia.org/wiki/File:Haemocytometer_side.svg. Copyright © 2006 by Ewen. Reprinted with permission

Fig. 2.6: Copyright © by ZEISS Microscopy (CC BY 2.0) at https://commons.wikimedia.org/wiki/File:Primo_Vert.jpg.

Fig. 2.7: Copyright © by Zeiss (CC BY 2.0) at https://commons.wikimedia.org/wiki/File:Microscope_Objective_Specifications.jpg.

■ Chapter 3

The Culture Environment

CHAPTER PURPOSE

This chapter discusses the importance of an ideal cell culture environment for maintaining mammalian cells in long-term cultures. Explanations are provided so that students can develop an appreciation for why these specific conditions are used in cell culture.

CHAPTER APPLICATION

The information in this chapter helps the reader gain a better understanding of the ideal conditions for mammalian cell cultures and troubleshoot, should problems arise. This chapter covers the importance of temperature and humidity levels in the incubator, osmolality of culture medium, buffering agents in the medium and the use of 5% and 10% carbon dioxide in incubators. The chapter explains in sufficient detail how the bicarbonate buffer system helps stabilize the pH. The chapter also discusses how cellular metabolic activity, or lack thereof, affects pH of the medium, cell growth and cell proliferation.

Temperature

Every cell type requires optimal culture conditions for optimal performance, be it for growth, proliferation, differentiation, or the production of recombinant molecules. Cellular functions are controlled by chemical reactions, driven by enzyme activity. Biochemical reactions include the transfer of ions between the intermediaries participating in these reactions. These reactions result in energy production, energy utilization, and transfer of ions between components in the reaction series to effect processes such as transport of molecules across various cellular compartments, functioning of cytoskeletal structures, duplication of cellular components, and cellular homeostasis. At lower than ideal temperature, enzyme efficiency diminishes and slows down cellular processes. Higher temperatures can destroy enzymes and negatively affect cell survival. Cells from different species perform better at different temperatures. For example, human and other mammalian cells perform optimally at 37 °C; chicken cells require an elevated temperature of 38.5 °C; insect cells perform best between 27 °C and 30 °C; and cells from cold-blooded animals perform best between 15 °C and 26 °C.

Osmolality

Osmolality is defined as the concentration of solutes in a solvent, expressed as the total number of solute particles per kilogram solvent. *Osmolarity* is often used interchangeably with "osmolality"; however, there are specific but subtle differences between the two terms. In physiological systems, "osmolality" is the more appropriate term to explain solute concentration. The physiological osmolality is approximately 285–295 milliosmoles per kilogram fluid (mOsm/kg). For cell cultures, an osmolality in the range of 260 to 320 mOsm/kg is used.

Selective permeability of the cell membrane restricts the movement of solutes across the membrane. Osmotic pull exerted by the solutes affect the movement of water across the membranes to equilibrate salt concentrations via a process termed *osmosis*. Use of hypotonic solutions can result in water moving into the cells, resulting in swelling and cell rupture. Conversely, use of hypertonic solutions can cause water to leave the cells, resulting in cell shrinkage and death. Cell culture media are formulated to be isotonic with the cells. It is also important to ensure that all buffers, wash solutions, and other reagents used to manipulate live cells are isotonic in nature.

Humidity

Incubation of cell culture plates and flasks at 37 °C poses the risk of evaporation of culture medium. In conditions of low or no humidity, the cultures can dry up within a few hours. To mitigate this risk, humidity between 95% and 100% is maintained in the incubators. A tray of sterile deionized water is kept in the incubator to maintain this level of humidity. It is important to monitor the incubator water level regularly and replenish as needed. Despite the precautions, a low level of evaporation occurs if the cultures are maintained in the incubator for longer than 5 to 7 days without media change.

Oxygen

Cell metabolism depends on the availability of dissolved oxygen in culture medium. Generally, cell cultures are maintained under ambient oxygen conditions (about 21% O_2). The ambient O_2 concentration is considered "normoxic". However, it is important to understand that body tissues experience much lower oxygen concentrations, ranging anywhere between a low of 4.6% O_2 in the brain to about 9.5% O_2 in the renal cortex (Muz et al., 2015), which is referred to as *physioxia*. Under pathological conditions, tissues may experience non-physiological levels of oxygen tension, termed *hypoxia*, generally seen in tumor tissues. In cell experimental studies, hypoxic incubators can be used to study the effects of low oxygen on cell growth or mimic tissue oxygenation conditions.

Carbon Dioxide, Sodium Bicarbonate, and pH Maintenance

The *pH*, or hydrogen potential, of a solution represents the measure of the degree of acidity or alkalinity of a solution on a pH scale ranging from 0 to 14. A pH value of 7 is considered neutral, a pH value below 7 indicates acidity, and a pH value above 7 indicates alkalinity. The pH is expressed as the negative log of hydrogen ion concentration

$$pH = -\log([H^+])$$

Mammalian cells thrive in the pH range of 7.0 to 7.7, with the physiological pH ranging between 7.3 and 7.4. Water molecules dissociate into H^+ and OH^- ions. At neutral pH, water contains approximately 10^{-7} moles/liter of H^+ ions (0.0000001 moles per liter). At physiological pH of 7.4, a solution contains approximately $10^{-7.4}$ moles/liter of H^+ ions (0.0000000389107 moles per liter). Two common buffer systems used in mammalian cell cultures are the bicarbonate and the HEPES buffer systems. Of the two, the bicarbonate buffer system is predominantly used in routine cell culture work. Sodium bicarbonate ($NaHCO_3$) is used as the source of bicarbonate ions in cell culture media. Media preparations are available with two different $NaHCO_3$ concentrations. Formulations containing 1.5 to 2.2 g/L are recommended for use with incubators set at 5% CO_2. Media formulations containing 3.7 g/L sodium bicarbonate are recommended for use with incubators set at 10% CO_2. In solution, $NaHCO_3$ dissociates to sodium (Na^+) and bicarbonate (HCO_3^-) ions. The HCO_3^- ions can react with free H^+ ions, thereby buffering the pH of the solution. The amount of CO_2 provided in the incubator (5% or 10%) is much higher than atmospheric CO_2 (0.03%). Following Henry's law, the high CO_2 content in the incubator results in the CO_2 dissolving in the culture medium to generate H^+ ions in the media (Figure 3.1). The H^+ and HCO_3^- ions reach an equilibrium to attain the physiological pH.

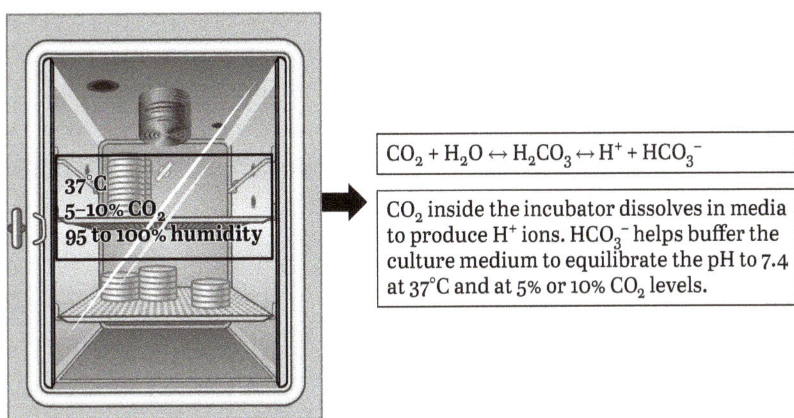

FIGURE 3.1 Achieving physiological pH in culture media inside the incubator.

The pH equilibrium can shift when actively dividing cells are present in the cultures. Metabolically active cells metabolize glucose to produce energy (ATP) for cellular activities. A byproduct of glucose metabolism is CO_2 (see Equation 1). The excess CO_2 resulting from the metabolic activity dissolves in the culture medium to generate excess H^+ ions (see Equation 2). The HCO_3^- ions from the $NaHCO_3$ in the medium acts to sequester the H^+ ions to buffer the pH. However, bicarbonate buffer is a weak buffer. Therefore, excessive cell proliferation can shift the pH to more acidic levels. Hence, to avoid pH related effects to cells, it is important to either subculture the cells or exchange the old medium with fresh medium periodically.

$$C_6H_{12}O_6 + 6O_2 \rightarrow ATP + 6CO_2 + 6H_2O \qquad \text{(Equation 1)}$$

$$CO_2 + H_2O \leftrightarrow H_2CO_3 \leftrightarrow H^+ + HCO_3^- \qquad \text{(Equation 2)}$$

Lack of CO_2 can negatively impact cell survival. If the CO_2 tank runs out of CO_2, the dynamics of pH maintenance in the culture medium are disturbed. Lack of CO_2 in the tanks will bring down the CO_2 levels in the incubator to atmospheric CO_2 levels (0.03%). Dissolved CO_2 will diffuse out of the medium, resulting in lower levels of H^+ in the medium. This shifts the pH of the medium to alkaline, severely affecting cell survival. Therefore, careful monitoring of CO_2 levels in the CO_2 tanks should be a routine aspect of cell culture, especially before weekends and holidays. In this context, it is important to note that gas exchange between the culture medium and the incubator environment is crucial to maintaining the pH. Placing the culture plates in tightly sealed secondary enclosures or under tight wraps around the lids or caps of plates or flasks will negatively impact cell growth.

An alternative to the bicarbonate buffer system is the HEPES [(4-(2-hydroxyethyl)-1-piperazineethane-sulfonic acid)] buffer at concentrations ranging from 10 to 25 mM HEPES. HEPES is a much stronger buffer that can maintain the pH at different temperatures and without the need for CO_2 supply. The two major drawbacks are that HEPES is comparatively more expensive and can be toxic to certain cell types at higher concentrations. The effect of interaction between the bicarbonate buffer, CO_2, and cellular metabolic activity inside a cell culture incubator is summarized in Table 3.1.

TABLE 3.1 Summary of the Effects of Excess CO_2 Production and CO_2 Depletion on Cell Cultures in CO_2 Incubators

Condition	What happens in the culture	Result
No cells in culture	No CO_2 production	pH remains stable at 7.4
Increased cell proliferation	Increased cellular metabolism	pH becomes acidic
	Increased CO_2 production	
	Reaction shifts to the right (see Equation 2)	
	Increased H^+ production	
CO_2 depletion in incubator (ambient CO_2)	Dissolved CO_2 escapes the medium	pH becomes alkaline
	Reaction shifts to the left (see Equation 2)	
	Reduction in H^+ ions	

Chapter Takeaways

The environment in which the cells are cultured can have a major impact on their performance. These factors include temperature, humidity levels in the incubator, osmolality of the culture medium, and O_2 and CO_2 levels. A better understanding of the importance of these parameters and their interplay helps a cell culturist troubleshoot any problems encountered in cell culture. A serious student should monitor the CO_2 and temperature settings on the incubator display as well as check the water level in the incubator daily. Cells are usually cultured under ambient oxygen; however, if special incubators are used for hypoxia or hyperoxia conditions, one should monitor the oxygen levels as well. The pH of the culture medium is affected by the interplay between the amount of bicarbonate in the medium, the CO_2 levels in the incubator (5% or 10%), the amount of CO_2 produced as a result of cellular metabolism, as well as depletion of CO_2 in the CO_2 tanks. Periodical subculturing and/or media change can help maintain the nutrient balance and proper cell density to help maintain a healthy cell culture.

References

Muz, B., de la Puente, P., Azab F., & Azab, A. K. (2015). The role of hypoxia in cancer progression, angiogenesis, metastasis, and resistance to therapy. *Hypoxia (Auckl)*, *3*, 83–92. https://www.doi.org/10.2147/HP.S93413. PMID: 27774485; PID: PMC5045092.

■ Chapter 4

Basal Culture Media and Media Supplements

CHAPTER PURPOSE

The process of cell culture involves the isolation of primary cells from fresh biopsies followed by culture in vitro as primary cells or the maintenance of continuous cultures from established cell lines. Cells cultured in vitro require the right mix of nutrients and growth factors for their robust growth and maintenance. Different cell types have different nutritional needs based on their physiology. The purpose of this chapter is to inform students the importance of understanding the composition of culture media for different cell types and the need to pay close attention to the differences between various formulations of the same basal media and other media supplements so that unintentional mistakes can be avoided.

CHAPTER APPLICATION

Students will learn the general composition of basal media and the supplements used to prepare complete media. Students will also gain a better understanding of the fundamentals of media preparation that should help them troubleshoot any issues observed in cell culture if the wrong media formulation is used. Students will learn to formulate their own complete media from basal media and high concentration stock of the supplements required for specific cell type(s) used in the experiment.

Culture Media Basics

The basic component of any cell culture medium is the *basal medium*. The basal medium is a cocktail of essential nutrients required to maintain cells in vitro. Different media formulations may contain different components suited for particular cell types.

Main Components of Basal Media

The following are the main components of basal media:

- **inorganic salts:** help regulate membrane potential and osmolality
- **amino acids:** the raw materials for the synthesis of proteins necessary for cell growth and maintenance. These amino acids are broadly categorized into two groups: (a) essential amino acids and (b) nonessential amino acids (NEAA).

    - **essential amino acids:** L-arginine, L-cystine, L-isoleucine, L-leucine, L-lysine, L-methionine, L-phenylalanine, L-threonine, L-tryptophan, L-histidine, L-tyrosine, and L-valine
    - **nonessential amino acids:** glycine, L-alanine, L-asparagine, L-aspartic acid, L-glutamic acid, L-proline, and L-serine

    All amino acids, except glycine, are L-amino acids. Cells are capable of synthesizing the nonessential amino acids on their own. Certain protocols suggest supplementing with NEAA because when the concentrations of these amino acids get low, glucose and glutamine consumption can increase and adversely affect cell growth.

- **vitamins:** cells do not synthesize vitamins. Vitamins function as cofactors and are essential for cellular growth and proliferation. The vitamin supplement includes D-calcium pantothenate, choline chloride, folic acid, i-inositol, nicotinamide, pyridoxal hydrochloride, riboflavin, and thiamine hydrochloride.
- **glucose:** it is the main carbohydrate source for energy production in the cells. Other sugars, such as galactose, fructose, or maltose, may be supplemented.
- **phenol red:** it is used as a pH indicator in cell culture media. Most basal media come supplemented with phenol red. When added to the culture media, it displays a red color when the medium is at physiologic pH, a yellow color at acidic pH, and a pink color at alkaline pH (Figure 4.1). While this feature is helpful for visual determination of pH, it is to be noted that phenol red has been shown to exhibit estrogenic activity and can affect cell behavior in estrogen responsive cells (Bukovsky, 2005; Grady et al., 1991; Walsh-Reitz et al., 1992). Media formulations without phenol red supplementation should be used to avoid effects of estrogen.

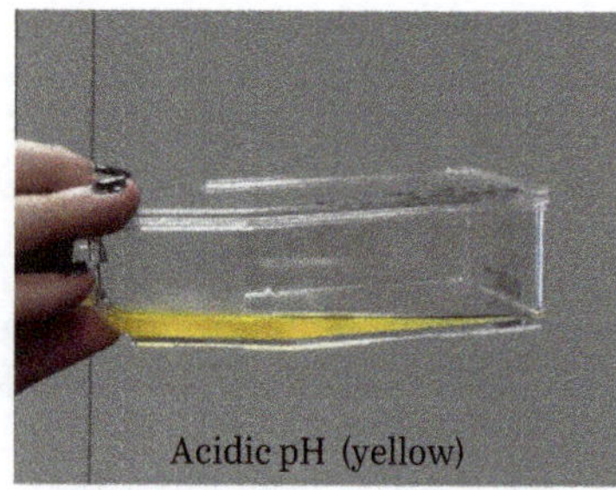

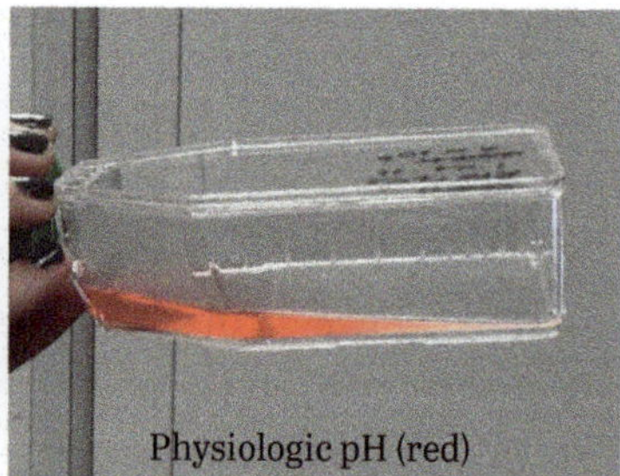

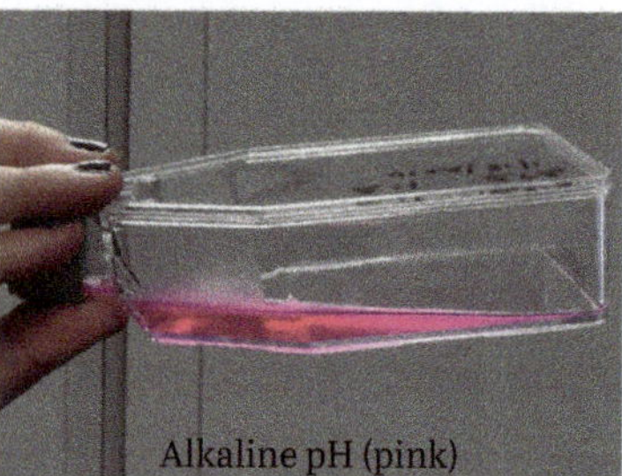

FIGURE 4.1 Phenol Red as a pH Indicator

- **buffering agents in culture medium:** biological processes are sensitive to pH changes. Therefore, maintaining the pH of culture medium within a range of 7.2 to 7.4 is critical for robust cell growth. The two most commonly used buffer systems in cell culture media are the bicarbonate buffer system and the HEPES buffer system; the bicarbonate buffer system being the most commonly used buffer system (see Chapter 3). HEPES belongs to a class of buffers called the "zwitterionic N-substituted aminosulfonic acids." It has a useful pH range of 6.8 to 8.2. HEPES meets all the basic requirements necessary for a biological buffer to function at physiological pH. The requirements include the pKa value being close to the desired pH value at 37 °C temperature and compatibility of the buffer with cell structures. Additionally, the buffer should not form complexes with macromolecules and metal ions, and it should not enter the cell and affect cellular activity. As a biological buffer, HEPES is used in the range of 10 mM to 25 mM. It is important to note that in animal cell cultures, HEPES is not used solely but supplemented with the bicarbonate buffer for extra buffering capacity when cell cultures are manipulated for extended periods outside the CO_2 incubator. For more information, please refer to Michl et al. (2019).

Media Supplements

A "complete medium" is prepared by supplementing basal medium with additional components necessary for cell growth and maintenance and for the prevention of the growth of contaminating organisms. Depending on the composition of the basal medium, all or some of the following supplements are added to the basal medium to prepare complete medium. For specialized medium, additional components may be added.

- **antibiotics:** Several antibiotics are used to supplement cell culture media to prevent growth of chance contaminants, such as bacteria, yeast, fungi, and mycoplasma. A combination of penicillin, streptomycin, and amphotericin B is routinely used in cell cultures. Antibiotics exert the following effects to prevent the growth of contaminating organisms:

  a. interference with cell wall synthesis
  b. inhibition of protein synthesis
  c. interference with nucleic acid synthesis
  d. inhibition of metabolic pathways
  e. inhibition of membrane function
  f. inhibition of ATP synthase

  One must be cognizant of the fact that antibiotics may negatively influence mammalian cell proliferation and cellular differentiation (Llobet et al., 2015). In such instances, cell culture without the addition of antibiotics may be warranted. Table 4.1 lists the commonly used antibiotics, their working concentrations, and their target organisms.

TABLE 4.1 Commonly Used Antibiotics in Cell Cultures

		Responsive microorganisms				
Reagent	**Working concentration**	**Gram (+) bacteria**	**Gram (-) bacteria**	**Yeast**	**Mold**	**Mycoplasma**
Amphotericin B	2.5 mg/L			+	+	
Ampicillin	100 mg/L	+	+			
Cephalothin	100 mg/L	+	+			
Dihydrostreptomycin	100 mg/L	+	+			
Erythromycin	100 mg/L	+	+			
Gentamicin sulfate	50 mg/L	+	+			+
Kanamycin	100 mg/L	+	+			+
Lincomycin HCl	100 mg/L	+				
Neomycin sulfate	50 mg/L	+	+			
Nystatin	50 mg/L			+	+	
Paromomycin sulfate	100 mg/L	+	+			
Penicillin G	100,000 U/L	+				
Polymyxin B sulfate	50 mg/L		+			
Spectinomycin	7.5-20 mg/L	+	+			
Streptomycin sulfate	100 mg/L	+	+			
Tetracycline hydrochloride	10 mg/L	+	+			
Tylosin tartrate	8 mg/L	+				+

Source: Merck KGaA, "Commonly Used Antibiotics in Cell Culture," https://www.sigmaaldrich.com/US/en/technical-documents/technical-article/cell-culture-and-cell-culture-analysis/cell-culture-troubleshooting/antibiotic-selector. Copyright © 2023 by Merck KGaA.

- **fetal bovine serum:** Serum is one of the most important and essential components of the complete medium. Serum is the fluid component of whole blood formed after the blood clots. It is a cocktail of thousands of proteins, polypeptides, fat, carbohydrates, growth factors, hormones, inorganic minerals, and other molecules (for a review, see Yang and Xiong, 2012). The history of supplementing serum in media formulations dates back to Harry Eagle (1955), who reported that the addition of a small amount of serum was needed to support cell growth. The widespread use of fetal bovine serum (FBS) in mammalian cell culture started after Puck et al. (1958) demonstrated that FBS stimulated cell growth in vitro. FBS contains higher concentrations of certain growth factors than serum from other species. The addition of 2% to 10% FBS takes care of most of the protein requirements for cultured cells. Higher or lower serum concentrations are used depending on the needs of individual cell types. FBS protects cells from large pH shifts, negative effects of proteases, shear forces, other toxic agents, and agents that would typically break up monolayers of adherent cells. Cell growth in the presence of FBS is rapid, consistent, and reproducible. Because of the low content of immunoglobulins and complement factors, FBS is preferred to other types of serum. Other types of bovine serum include neonatal bovine serum, newborn calf serum, bovine calf serum, and adult serum (Table 4.2). Human, horse, goat, donkey, and chicken sera are also used for specific purposes. The typical composition of serum is provided in Table 4.3.

TABLE 4.2 Types of Bovine Serum

Serum type	Common abbreviation	Age at collection
Fetal bovine serum	FBS or FCS	Fetuses of healthy dams
Neonatal bovine serum	NBS	Less than 10 days, having not suckled
Newborn calf serum	NBCS	Less than 20 days
Bovine calf serum	BCS	20 days to 12 months
Donor calf serum	DCS	12 months or older from controlled donor herds
Adult bovine serum	ABS	12 months or older, having been deemed healthy after ante- and/or post-mortem inspection

Source: Bio-Techne, "Types of Bovine Serum," https://resources.rndsystems.com/images/site/rnd-systems-fbs-br3.pdf.

TABLE 4.3 Typical Composition of Serum

Serum component grouping	Individual components
Serum proteins	Albumin
	Globulins (e.g., immunoglobulins, IgG)
	α antitrypsin (protease inhibitor)
	α2 macroglobulin (protease inhibitor)
Transport proteins	Transferrin
	Transcortin
	α1 lipoprotein
	β1 lipoprotein
Attachment and spreading factors	Fibronectin
	Laminin
	Serum spreading factor
Enzymes	Lactate dehydrogenase
	Alkaline phosphatase
	Y-glutamyl transferase
	Alanine aminotransferase (ALT/GPT)
	Aspartate aminotransferase (AST/GOT)
Hormones	Insulin
	Glucagon
	Corticosteroids
	Vasopressin
	Thyroid hormones
	Parathyroid hormone
	Growth hormone
	Pituitary glandotropic factors
	Prostaglandins

(Continued)

TABLE 4.3 *(Continued)*

Serum component grouping	Individual components
Growth factors and cytokines	Epidermal growth factor (EGF)
	Fibroblast growth factor (FGF)
	Nerve growth factor (NGF)
	Endothelial cell growth factor (ECGF)
	Platelet-derived growth factor (PDGF)
	Insulin-like growth factors (IGFs)
	Interleukins
	Interferons
	Transforming growth factors (TGFs)
Fatty acids and lipids	Free and protein-bound fatty acids
	Triglycerides
	Phospholipids
	Cholesterol
	Ethanolamine
	Phosphatidylethanolamine
Vitamins and trace elements	Retinol/retinoic acid (vitamin A)
	Thiamine, riboflavin, pyridoxine/pyridoxalphosphate, cobalamin, folic acid, niacinamide/nicotinic acid, panthotenic acid, and biotin (vitamin B)
	Ascorbic acid (vitamin C)
	a-tocopherol (vitamin E)
	Selenium, iron, zinc, copper, cobalt, chromium, iodine, fluorine, manganese, molybdenum, vanadium, nickel, and tin
Carbohydrates	Glucose
	Galactose
	Fructose
	Mannose
	Ribose
	Glycolytic metabolites
Nonprotein nitrogens	Urea
	Purine/pyrimidines
	Polyamines
	Creatinine
	Amino acids

- **sodium pyruvate:** Sodium pyruvate is an optional component in cell culture media. It functions as a carbon source in addition to glucose. It is supplemented at a final concentration of 1 mM to prepare complete medium. Media formulations with and without sodium pyruvate supplementation are available.
- **L-glutamine or L-alanyl-L-glutamine:** L-glutamine is an essential amino acid supplemented in most cell culture media. It is highly unstable in solutions at physiological pH and can break down into ammonia and pyroglutamate. It is stable for only about 1 week in solutions stored at 4 °C. Ammonia resulting from the degradation of L-glutamine can become toxic to cells. Degradation depends on the pH and temperature. Heeneman et al. (1993) reported that commercially available cell culture media supplemented with L-glutamine contained varying levels of ammonia, up to 1,000 μM. A stabilized form of glutamine, a dipeptide named L-alanyl-L-glutamine, is an analog of L-glutamine. This component remains stable in solution and allows for extended cell culturing with less frequent media changes. This benefit is attributed to the fact that L-alanyl-L-glutamine is broken down only after cellular uptake of the dipeptide, as opposed to spontaneous breakdown during storage. Cell cultures are usually supplemented with 2 to 4 mM L-glutamine or L-alanyl-L-glutamine. Media formulations with and without L-glutamine or L-alanyl-L-glutamine supplementation are available.

Serum Replacements and Serum Substitutes

Even though FBS is a crucial component of cell culture medium, it suffers from several disadvantages, including (a) batch-to-batch variability, (b) risk of potentially harmful microbiological agents, (c) concerns related to the ethics of using inhumane methods of serum harvesting, and (d) economic concerns due the high cost involved in procurement and processing of the product (Bauman et al., 2018). Therefore, use of serum alternatives and serum substitutes have been proposed, especially in the development of cell therapy products for human applications. Examples of serum substitutes include human platelet lysate, human serum, human recombinant proteins, recombinant growth factors and hormones, synthetic peptides, and bovine ocular fluid. Media prepared using serum and alternatives to serum can be broadly classified as (a) animal serum based, (b) serum free, (c) xeno-free, (d) animal component free, (e) protein free, and (f) chemically defined media (Table 4.4). Because of the ethical issues associated with the use of animal serum, a collaborative effort between the Dutch 3Rs-Centre ULS and Animal Free Research UK launched a Fetal Calf Serum-Free database (https://fcs-free.org/). The database was launched in 2017 to educate scientists and researchers about the ethical issues associated with the use of animal serum and to provide information about a range of commercially available serum-free media and serum alternatives for cell culture.

TABLE 4.4 Classification of Serum and Serum Substitutes in Cell Culture Media

Term	Definition	Advantages
Serum containing media	Media containing animal or human serum; additional growth factors are sometimes supplemented	Contains growth factors
		Helps cell attachment
		Helps to buffer the pH
Serum free media	Media not containing either serum or unprocessed plasma; additional growth factors may be supplemented	Batch-to-batch consistency
		Provides better control over culture conditions
		Lower risk of contamination with bacteria, fungi or viruses
Xeno-free media	Media containing components derived from nonanimal sources; however, xeno-free media can contain human-derived supplements	Eliminates variability due to undefined animal components
		Improved consistency in both performance and quality
		No risk of microbial contaminants
Animal component–free media	Media not containing either animal- or human-derived components	Batch-to-batch consistency
		Traceability of components
		Simplifies compliance with regulatory guidelines
Chemically defined media	Media not containing proteins, growth factors, hydrolysates, or components of unknown composition; may contain a mixture of recombinant materials (proteins, hormones, cytokines, and/or growth factors)	Batch-to-batch consistency
		Elimination of factors that may interfere with hormones or growth factors when studying their interaction with cells
		No risk of microbial contaminants
Protein-free media	Media containing no proteins but often containing hydrolyzed proteins	Batch-to-batch consistency
		Facilitates downstream protein purification and processing

Adapted from Ohad Karnieli, et al., "Table 1" from "Classification of Serum and Serum Substitutes in Cell Culture Media," *Cytotherapy*, vol. 19, no. 2, p. 159.

Selecting the Right Medium for Your Culture Needs

There are several commercially available basal media for use with different cell types. Each formulation comes with a different composition as far as supplementation is concerned. For example, the formulations of DMEM may vary in their amount of glucose, L-glutamine, sodium pyruvate, sodium bicarbonate, HEPES, and other components (Table 4.5). Therefore, one must be cognizant of the differences between formulations for the same basal media and choose the right media for specific applications. The most commonly used basal media are listed below:

a. Eagle's minimal essential medium (MEM)
b. Dulbecco's modified Eagle's medium (DMEM)
c. Iscove's basic DMEM (IMDM)
d. Roswell Park Memorial Institute medium (RPMI-1640)
e. Medium 199/109
f. Ham's F-10/Ham's F-12
g. McCoy's 5A

While choosing the basal media for cell culture needs, one should pay close attention to the composition of the particular basal media. For example, different DMEM formulations with different catalog numbers may vary in the amount of a particular ingredient or the presence or absence of one or more ingredients (Table 4.5). For example, cells that require high glucose may not perform well with product #10-014, which has a low glucose content. Product numbers 17-205, 17-207, and 15-013 require L-glutamine supplementation. While product #10-027 contains both $NaHCO_3$ and HEPES as buffering agents, product numbers 50-003 and 50-013 provide the flexibility of adding the desired buffering agent depending on the customer's needs. Sodium pyruvate supplementation is required for 10-027, 17-207, and 50-013 if the cells require sodium pyruvate supplementation. Product numbers 17-205, 50-003, and 50-013 do not contain phenol red and, hence, will not exhibit color shift in the media with changing pH. It is, therefore, critical to understand the differences in media composition, as this allows one to troubleshoot if the cell growth dynamics show deviation from the norm.

TABLE 4.5 Differences in Composition of Ingredients in DMEM Basal Media (Based on Corning products)

Ingredients (DMEM)	Corning catalog number							
	10-013	**10-014**	**10-027**	**17-205**	**17-207**	**15-013**	**50-003**	**50-013**
D-glucose	High	Low	High	High	None	High	High	High
L-glutamine	Yes	Yes	Yes	No	No	No	Yes	Yes
Sodium pyruvate	Yes	Yes	No	Yes	No	Yes	Yes	No
Sodium bicarbonate	Yes	Yes	Yes	Yes	Yes	Yes	No	No
HEPES	No	No	Yes	No	No	No	No	No
Phenol red	Yes	Yes	Yes	No	Yes	Yes	No	No

Corning Incorporated, "Differences in Composition of Ingredients in DMEM Basal Media," https://www.corning.com/catalog/cls/documents/formulations/CLS-CG-BR-001-DMEM-Formulations.pdf.

Preparing Basal Media From Powdered Media

Some labs prefer to prepare their own basal media from powdered media, primarily due to the low cost, especially if the lab uses large volumes of media for their daily needs. The use of powdered media has the advantage of letting a researcher prepare small or large volumes of media or prepare 5x or 10x concentrated media, as necessary. To prepare basal media solution, powdered media is dissolved in sterile water and pH adjustments are made per the manufacturer's instructions. The solution may require additional glucose, sodium bicarbonate, or HEPES or other components as the protocol demands. The final basal medium should be filter sterilized using 0.22-micron filters. Media should never be sterilized using autoclaving as it can denature and inactivate proteins and cause charring of glucose when exposed to elevated temperatures.

Preparing Complete Media

While preparing complete media or any reagent from individual components, it is a good lab practice to create a table listing the individual components with their stock concentrations, final desired concentrations, vendor name, and catalog numbers. This allows one to backtrack and troubleshoot any problems very effectively. The most common mistake encountered in a laboratory with a "protocol-based" approach is that the protocols list only the components and their respective volumes or weights, without information about the specific details of the products. Understanding the products and their specifications is key to successful experimentation (Table 4.6).

Keeping track of the details of reagents helps troubleshoot problems. DMEM basal media #15-013 (Corning) does not contain L-Glutamine. Failure to supplement the complete medium with L-glutamine or L-alanyl-L-glutamine can result in poor cell growth. Use of DMEM basal media (product #10-014, Corning) instead of 15-013 could lead to reduced cell proliferation due to the lower glucose content in product #10-014. Use of basal media #10-027 (Corning) requires sodium pyruvate supplementation. In cases where additional components are added, the volume of the basal medium should be adjusted to prepare the desired final volume of complete medium.

TABLE 4.6 Complete Media Composition Chart

Order of addition	Component	Catalog #	Supplier	Stock concentration	Final concentration	Volume
1	DMEM basal medium	15-013	Corning	N/A	Up to 100 ml	88 ml
2	Glutamax	35050061	Thermo Fisher	200 mM	2 mM	1 ml
3	Penicillin/Streptomycin	15140122	Thermo Fisher	100X	1X	1 ml
4	FBS	S11150	Atlanta Bio	100%	1X	10 ml
	Total volume					100 ml

Nonmedia Reagents

Nonmedia reagents include trypsin, for dissociating cells from the culture plate; balanced salt solutions, such as phosphate buffered saline (PBS); Dulbecco's phosphate-buffered saline (DPBS); Hanks' Balanced Salt Solution (HBSS), for rinsing cells; and sterile water for preparing reagents.

Trypsin

Trypsin, a mixture of proteases derived from porcine pancreas, is a commonly used cell dissociating agent. Trypsin is used to dissociate and lift cells off the culture plate during subculturing. Trypsin comes in powder form or in ready-to-use format that may or may not be supplemented with ethylenediaminetetraacetic acid (EDTA) and phenol red. EDTA is a chelating agent that can bind metal ions such as calcium, magnesium, lead, and iron. The presence of calcium and magnesium in the media or buffers can inhibit the protease activity of trypsin. EDTA helps bind any residual calcium and magnesium ions and weakens the cell attachment to the plates, thus allowing trypsin to work more efficiently. The composition of trypsin solution used for cell dissociation is 0.05% trypsin with 0.53 mM EDTA. Trypsin activity is optimal at 37 °C. Trypsin treatment should be limited to the minimum time required to dissociate the cells. Since it is a protease, longer incubation times can damage the cells by stripping the cell surface proteins and eventually killing the cells. Complete medium containing FBS or a small amount of pure FBS (0.05%) should be added to the plate after trypsin treatment to neutralize trypsin activity. This prevents further protease activity and cell damage during subsequent cell processing steps. The presence of FBS after trypsin treatment also help neutralize the static charge in the centrifuge tubes. Failure to add FBS after trypsinization can make the cells adhere to the walls of the centrifuge tube resulting in major cell loss.

In experiments where the use of trypsin is not recommended, trypsin alternatives may be used. Enzymatic alternatives include collagenase, dispase, or commercially available formulations such as Tryple (recombinant porcine trypsin), Accutase, Accumax, Detachin, and HyrTryp. Nonenzymatic trypsin alternatives include EDTA (0.5 mM) and EDTA/EGTA mixtures (1 mM each).

Note that prior to trypsinizing cells, the plate should be rinsed with a buffered saline such as PBS or DPBS without Ca^{++} and Mg^{++} to remove any residual complete medium and Ca^{++} and Mg^{++} from the plate. The presence of alpha-1-antitrypsin in the FBS can inhibit trypsin activity (Stockley, 2015). Therefore, rinsing with a Ca^{++}/Mg^{++}-free buffer solution helps remove these inhibitory agents from the plate.

Buffered Salt Solutions

Phosphate buffered saline (PBS), Dulbecco's phosphate-buffered saline (pH 7.4, with and without Ca^{++}/ $Mg^{++)}$ or Hank's balanced salt solution (HBSS) are used in cell culture work for rinsing and resuspending cells (see buffer composition in Appendix III). For cell dissociation, buffers free of divalent cations Ca^{++} and Mg^{++} should be used for reasons explained above.

Chapter Takeaways

The composition of culture media is the most critical factor in the maintenance of healthy cell cultures. Therefore, a good understanding of the needs of specific cell types and the proper selection of suitable culture media is critical. For example, the osteoblastic cell line 7F2 (ATCC, CRL-12557) requires alpha-MEM medium supplemented with 10% FBS, L-glutamine, and sodium pyruvate <u>without</u> ribonucleosides and deoxyribonucleosides, while the preosteoblastic cell line MC3T3-E1 clone 4 (ATCC, CRL-2593) requires alpha-MEM medium supplemented with 10% FBS, L-glutamine, and sodium pyruvate without ascorbic acid but <u>with</u> ribonucleosides and deoxyribonucleosides. The growth dynamics of cells grown in Corning DMEM cat #10-013 and cat #10-014 will be different because of the difference in glucose content. Similarly, formulations with and without specific components, for e.g., L-glutamine, sodium pyruvate, sodium bicarbonate, HEPES etc. are available (Table 4.5 and Appendix IV). Students should learn to pay attention to these product details, making it a habit as part of their lab etiquette.

A good lab practice while preparing complete media is to create a table listing the basal media, stock concentrations of supplements, and volumes used of each component in the final complete media mix, as shown in Table 4.6. Most importantly, students must understand the "final concentrations" of individual components (for e.g., 5% or 10% FBS and 2mM or 4mM L-glutamine) rather than mere volumes or weights of components. This habit serves the student better in preparing the final reagent mixture more efficiently and effectively. Table 4.7 helps the student troubleshoot should there be problems associated with a reagent. With regard to FBS, variations due to different manufacturers and different batches (even from the same manufacturer) can be problematic. While ordering new FBS, it is best to evaluate multiple batches of FBS to determine the batch number that works best for your cells. To conclude, a cell culturist should know not just what to use but also why certain components are needed for optimal cell growth.

Troubleshooting Guide

Students must understand not only the "what" and "how" of a protocol but also the "why" of every single aspect of the procedure to effectively troubleshoot issues if and when they arise in the experiments. Table 4.7 lists some of the most common issues encountered in cell culture labs.

TABLE 4.7 Troubleshooting Cell Culture Problems

Problem	Possible reason	Remedy
The basal media is colorless.	The product comes without phenol red supplementation.	None. If desired, phenol red may be added to medium at a concentration of 15 mg per liter.
Cells do not detach after prolonged trypsinization.	The trypsin has expired.	Use new trypsin.
	The wrong wash buffer containing Ca^{++}/Mg^{++} was used.	Aspirate the trypsin, and rinse with a wash buffer without Ca^{++}/Mg^{++}. Repeat trypsinization.
	The plate was not incubated at 37 °C.	Incubation at lower temperatures can delay the effectiveness of trypsinization. Incubate the plate at 37 °C.
There is poor cell survival after trypsinization.	Trypsin concentration is too high.	Correct the issue for the procedure next time.
	Prolonged trypsin treatment.	Monitor the cells for effectiveness of trypsinization. Use the minimal time required for cell detachment.
	The incubation temperature was too high.	Incubate the plate at 37 °C.
	A hypotonic solution was used to rinse the cells (e.g., water instead of PBS or DPBS).	Use buffered balanced salt solutions, such as PBS/DPBS without Ca^{++}/Mg^{++}.

Problem	Possible reason	Remedy
Cell yield is low after trypsinization and centrifugation.	Complete medium containing FBS was not added to the cell suspension after trypsinization. Static charge in the centrifuge tube can result in cells adhering to the walls of the tube, resulting in reduced cell yield.	Cells that adhered to the sides of the tube cannot be retrieved. Correct the issue for the procedure next time.
	Most of the cells are still on the plate.	Rinse the plate with wash buffer without Ca^{++}/Mg^{++}. Re-trypsinize the cells, collect them, and centrifuge again.
	There was no proper centrifugation, or the centrifuge failed to function.	Repeat centrifugation.
	The problem persists after repeated centrifugation.	The g-force may be low. Set the g-force between 200 g and 250 g (not RPM).
There is poor cell survival after centrifugation.	The g-force was too high.	Adjust the g-force to between 200 g and 250 g (not RPM).
There is poor cell growth with the use of a new culture medium.	There are low concentrations of essential ingredients in the medium.	Check the catalog number of the basal medium to ensure that it contains the ingredients necessary for cell growth. If needed, supplement the medium with the missing or low concentration ingredients (e.g., glucose, L-glutamine, sodium pyruvate, FBS, or other growth factors recommended for the cell line).
	Wrong basal media was used (e.g., RPMI-1640 instead of DMEM for fibroblast cultures).	Prepare the right culture medium.
The culture is contaminated with microorganisms.	Antibiotic and/or antimycotic supplements were not used.	Prepare fresh complete medium with antibiotic and antimycotic supplements.
	Antibiotic and/or antimycotic supplements have expired.	Use new antibiotic and or antimycotic supplements.
The amount of medium has diminished drastically, or the plate looks dry.	Evaporation of media occurred because there was not enough moisture inside the incubator.	Add enough sterile water to the tray to keep the moisture at 95% to 100% in the incubator.
The medium looks clear but the color of the medium is yellow.	Excessive cell growth.	Adjust the initial cell seeding number or passage the cells earlier.

(Continued)

TABLE 4.7 *(Continued)*

Problem	Possible reason	Remedy
The medium looks turbid and the color of the medium is yellow.	This is an indication of possible contamination with microorganisms.	Check the plate under the microscope for possible contamination. If contaminated, do not bring the plate inside the hood. Do not put the plate back in the incubator. Bring the culture plate to the sink, add 10% bleach to the culture for overnight treatment, and then discard. Start a new culture.
		Check the original culture media stock for turbidity/bacterial growth. If necessary, discard the media stock and prepare fresh medium.
		Check other cultures for contamination where the same medium was used.
		Review aseptic procedures, and take corrective actions as needed.
The color of the medium is deep pink, and the cells are dead.	The incubator has run out of CO_2.	Replace the CO_2 tank. Make it a practice to monitor CO_2 levels periodically.
There is water condensation on the interior glass door of incubator.	The glass door is not heated.	Repair or replace the glass door.

References

Bauman, E., Granja, P. L., & Barrias, C. C. (2018). Fetal bovine serum-free culture of endothelial progenitor cells-progress and challenges. *Journal of Tissue Engineering and Regenerative Medicine*, *12*(7),1567–78. https://www.doi.org/10.1002/term.2678. Epub 2018 May 30. PMID: 29701896.

Brunner, D., Frank, J., Appl, H., Schöffl, H., Pfaller, W., & Gstraunthaler, G. (2010). Serum-free cell culture: The serum-free media interactive online database. *ALTEX*, *27*(1), 5362. https://www.doi.org/10.14573/altex.2010.1.53. PMID: 20390239.

Bukovsky, A., Svetlikova, M., & Caudle, M. R. (2005). Oogenesis in cultures derived from adult human ovaries. *Reproductive Biology and Endocrinology*, *3*(17). https://www.doi.org/10.1186/1477-7827-3-17. PMID: 15871747; PMCID: PMC1131924.

Grady, L. H., Nonneman, D. J., Rottinghaus, G. E., & Welshons, W. V. (1991). pH-dependent cytotoxicity of contaminants of phenol red for MCF-7 breast cancer cells. *Endocrinology*, *129*(6), 3321–30. https://www.doi.org/10.1210/endo-129-6-3321. PMID: 1954908.

Heeneman, S., Deutz, N. E., & Buurman, W. A. (1993). The concentrations of glutamine and ammonia in commercially available cell culture media. *Journal of Immunological Methods*, *166*(1), 85–91. https://www.doi.org/10.1016/0022-1759(93)90331-z. PMID: 8228290.

Karnieli, O., Friedner, O. M., Allickson, J. G., Zhang, N., Jung, S., Fiorentini, D., Abraham, E., Eaker, S. S., Yong, T. K., Chan, A., Griffiths, S., Wehn, A. K., Oh, S., Karnieli, O. (2017). A consensus introduction to serum replacements and serum-free media for cellular therapies. *Cytotherapy*, *19*(2), 155–169. https://www.doi.org/10.1016/j.jcyt.2016.11.011. PMID: 28017599.

Llobet, L., Montoya, J., López-Gallardo, E., & Ruiz-Pesini, E. (2015). Side effects of culture media antibiotics on cell differentiation. *Tissue Eng Part C Methods*, *21*(11), 1143–7. https://www.doi.org/10.1089/ten.TEC.2015.0062. PMID: 26037505.

Michl, J., Park, K. C., & Swietach, P. (2019). Evidence-based guidelines for controlling pH in mammalian live-cell culture systems. *Communications Biology—Nature*, 2(144). https://www.doi.org/10.1038/s42003-019-0393-7. PMID: 31044169; PMCID: PMC6486606.

Puck, T. T., Cieciura, S. J., & Robinson, A. (1958). Genetics of somatic mammalian cells: Long-term cultivation of euploid cells from human and animal subjects. *Journal of Experimental Medicine*, *108*(6), 945–56. https://www.doi.org/10.1084/jem.108.6.945. PMID: 13598821; PMCID: PMC2136918.

Stockley, R. A. (2015). The multiple facets of alpha-1-antitrypsin. *Annals of Translational Medicine*, *3*(10), 130. https://www.doi.org/10.3978/j.issn.2305-5839.2015.04.25. PMID: 26207223; PMCID: PMC4486914.

Walsh-Reitz, M. M., & Toback, F. G. (1992). Phenol red inhibits growth of renal epithelial cells. *American Journal of Physiology-Renal Physiology*, *262*, F687–F691.

Yang, Z., & Xiong, H.-R. (2012). Culture conditions and types of growth media for mammalian cells. *Biomedical tissue culture*. https://www.doi.org/10.5772/52301

Chapter 5

Important Concepts in Cell Culture

CHAPTER PURPOSE

The purpose of this chapter is to educate students on some important concepts in cell culture, such as classification of cell types, the applications and limitations of cell culture in research, and clinical applications of cell culture. The concepts explained in this chapter provide students with a breadth of knowledge they can apply to their cell culture techniques, understanding sources of error, and troubleshoot when problems arise.

CHAPTER APPLICATION

Students of cell culture must develop an understanding of the source of cells and the types of cells they are experimenting with. One must also learn to use the right cells to achieve their experimental objectives. For instance, research focused on evaluating the effect of a new drug against human lung cancer should use cell lines derived from that particular tumor type. Developing tissue engineered products, such as an organoid, may require primary cells capable of growing in a 3D culture system. Studies involving skeletal muscle disease require skeletal muscle model, not smooth or cardiac muscle model. Students should have a thorough understanding of the differences between primary cells, established cell lines, finite versus continuous cell lines, spontaneously generated cell lines, transformed cell lines, immortalized cell lines, stem cells (natural or induced), etc. An important concept such as the "Hayflick limit" explains the importance of distinguishing passage number versus cellular age. Other concepts covered include 2D versus 3D culture; biological contamination; and, most importantly, the dangers of cross-culture contamination and why researchers should be cognizant of the devastation it can cause,

Concept #1: The "Hayflick Limit"

Until about the early 1960s, the prevailing notion amongst cell biologists was that animal cells have unlimited proliferative capacity. This was in large part due to the influence of the studies of Alexis Carrel, who claimed to have developed an immortal chick heart tissue culture that his lab was able to maintain for more than 34 years from 1912 to 1946 (Carrel, 1912; Ebeling, 1922, Witkowski, 1980). It was the pioneering work by Leonard Hayflick in the 1960s that challenged the notion of the "infinite lifespan" of primary cells. *Hayflick limit* defines the concept behind "cellular ageing" of normal diploid cells (Hayflick & Moorhead, 1961; Hayflick, 1965). According to the Hayflick limit, normal diploid human cells can replicate only 40 to 60 times before the cells attain replicative senescence and stop dividing (see Figure 5.1) As it happens with new discoveries that go against prevailing beliefs, Hayflick's idea was rejected in the early days. It was not until the 1990s that his hypothesis was accepted by the mainstream scientists (Hayflick, 1998). Hayflick limit is an established fact today. Another major contribution by Hayflick include the development of immortalized cells for vaccine production that led to the birth of the biotechnology industry.

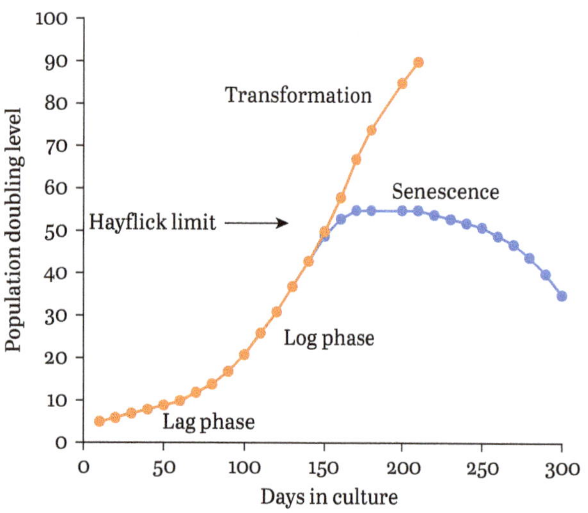

FIGURE 5.1 The Hayflick Limit in Normal Diploid Human Cells. It is characterized by the early lag phase, a log phase, replicative senescence, and then eventual cell death. Notice the senescence occurring at about 52 population doublings. Cells escaping the Hayflick limit undergo transformation and develop into cell lines with unlimited proliferative capacity.

Concept #2: Primary Cells and Cell Lines

Cell culture has become an indispensable tool in basic cell biology, biomedical and clinical research applications, and biomanufacturing. Some of the basic cell biology research areas include the study of cell cycle control, cell–cell interaction, cell-matrix interaction, cellular and organelle physiology, gene function, cancer biology, virology, and development of gene therapy techniques, to name a few. In the biomedical and clinical applications, cells have been used extensively as model systems for studying disease pathologies, drug testing, characterizing cancer cells, determining the role of chemicals, viruses, and radiation in cancer development, biomanufacturing vaccines, monoclonal antibodies, and stem cell therapies (Verma et al., 2020).

Terms used to define different cell types:

- **primary cells:** Every cell or cell line used in cell culture studies originated from biopsies, resected tissues from surgical procedures, or embryos. Cells from the tissues are isolated by various means, such as (a) physical disaggregation, (b) enzymatic digestion and chemical treatment (collagenase, dispase, DNase, trypsin, EDTA, EGTA), or (c) primary explant techniques (Richter *et al.*, 2021; Shannon *et al.*, 2022; Durkin *et al.*, 2013; Nejaddehbashi *et al.*, 2019). Primary cells are derived directly from an individual and expanded *in vitro* until they reach high confluence in the original cell culture vessel. Primary cells retain the original characteristics of the tissue from which they were derived.
- **primary cell line with limited lifespan:** Once the primary cells reach confluence in the original plate, the cells must be subcultured to new plates. Once the cells are transferred to new plates, they are called "primary cell lines with finite lifespan." These cells replicate until they reach the Hayflick limit, achieve replicative senescence, and die off.
- **continuous cell line with unlimited lifespan:** In rare circumstances, cells from primary cell lines undergo a process called "transformation." Transformed cells can be defined as cells that escaped the normal cell cycle controls and senescence with the potential for unlimited replication. At this point, they are called "continuous cell lines with unlimited lifespan." Transformation may happen spontaneously, induced using chemicals or viruses, or by making stable transgenic cell lines constitutively expressing the gene for telomerase reverse transcriptase (TERT).
- **cell strain:** These are subpopulations of cells either derived from positive selection of cells from a culture; or clones of cells expanded following single-cell isolation.

Concept #3: Passage Number and Population Doubling Limit and Population Doubling Level (PDL)

Distinction between passage number and PDL

- **passage number:** The "passage number" is the number of times cells have been subcultured—that is, the number of times cells have been harvested from one plate and moved into a new plate. The higher the passage number is, the older the cells are. Factors such as seeding density and frequency of subculturing can affect cell ageing. Therefore, passage number should be used only as a guide, not as an absolute definition of the "true age" of cells.
- **population doubling limit and population doubling level (PDL):** The "population doubling limit" (PDL) represents the number of times cells have doubled at the "population level." The population doubling limit is relevant in the case of primary cells because of their limited lifespan (Hayflick limit). Population doubling limit, therefore, reflects the "true age" of primary cells. A slightly different concept—the "population doubling level"—refers to the number of population doublings an established cell line undergoes over a period of time. Depending on the seeding density and frequency of subculturing, cell populations may undergo various levels of doubling within a single passage. Therefore, only PDL is the true representation of the **age** of cells. Hence,

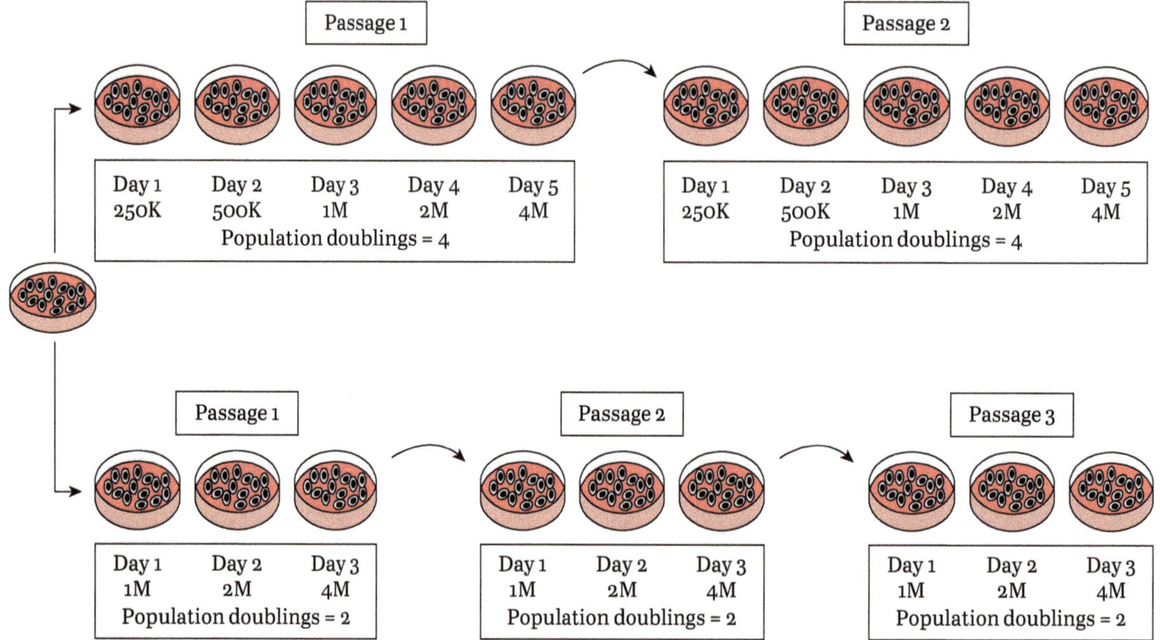

FIGURE 5.2 Passage Number vs. Population Doubling Limit (PDL) in Primary Cells. Assume that (a) these cells double once every 24 hours and (b) cells are ready to be subcultured when the confluency reaches 4 million cells in the plate. Notice that in the top half of the figure, due to the lower initial plating density (250,000 cells), cells undergo four population doublings in one passage before reaching subculture confluency. In the bottom half, due to the higher initial plating density (1 million cells), cells undergo only two population doublings in one passage before reaching subculture confluency. This difference becomes cumulative in subsequent passages. Therefore, cells from the top half will reach the Hayflick limit in fewer passages than cells in the bottom half.

one must diligently track the PDL of cells to ascertain their true age. While designing experiments with primary cells, care must be taken to consider the age of cells rather than passage number. In experiments, comparison of cellular activity of similar PDLs is more meaningful. The importance of PDL tracking is illustrated in Figure 5.2.

Concept #4: Cell Culture for Research vs. Tissue Engineering

A serious student of cell culture must have a thorough comprehension of the differences between cell culture for research purposes and for tissue engineering or cell therapy. Primary cells or cell lines representing a tissue type can be useful in elucidating the biology of that cell or tissue type using well-thought-out experimental designs. However, the approaches and preferences regarding tissue engineering and cell therapy are vastly different from cell biology research. Cells used for transplantation must meet specific requirements. The cells should be (a) immune compatible (b) nontumorigenic,

TABLE 5.1 Cell Source for Cell-Based Therapies

Cell source	Examples	Cell engraftment
Autologous	Hematopoietic stem cells, T cells	Potentially permanent
Allogeneic	Mesenchymal stem cells, Natural killer cells, B cells	Transient engraftment
Xenogeneic	Porcine pancreatic islet cells, choroid plexus cells	Transient engraftment
Sequestered cells (encapsulation or device)	β-Cells, Retinal pigment epithelial cells, hepatocytes	User-defined engraftment
Genetically modified non-immunogenic cells	Universal cells	Potentially permanent

Source: Bashor et al, 2022, "Cell Source for Cell-based Therapies" from "Engineering the Next Generation of Cell-based Therapeutics," *Nature Reviews Drug Discovery*, vol. 21, no. 9. Copyright © 2022 by Springer Nature.

and (c) functionally equivalent to the target tissue. Cells for tissue engineering and cell therapy are derived from autologous, allogeneic, or xenogeneic sources. Use of genetically modified nonimmunogenic cells is another option (Bashor et al., 2022). Table 5.1 lists the sources of cells and their utility in cell-based therapies. Another important consideration is the age of cells. Even though autologous cells are desirable due to their ability to avoid graft versus host disease, most patients waiting for tissue and organ transplantation are elderly people. Primary cells derived from older patients can be problematic due to the "age" of these cells, because they reach senescence more quickly, making the prospect of generating millions of cells from a tissue biopsy challenging (Khorraminejad-Shirazi et al., 2019). The problem becomes more acute if an emergency intervention is warranted. If time is not a major concern, generating induced pluripotent stem cells (iPSCs) from older patients is an alternative approach. However, one must consider the lower efficiency in generating iPSCs from older patients (Wen et al., 2013). Despite the low efficiency, reprogrammed cells from the elderly patients exhibited suppression of the senescent genes (Ohmine et al., 2012), pointing to their utility as a promising approach.

Concept #5: 2D Culture vs. 3D Culture

The traditional method of cell culture, *2D culture*, involves culturing cells on polystyrene culture dishes in a 2D environment or in suspension cultures. It must be appreciated that these cells originated from a 3D environment and were surrounded by multiple cell types within unique microenvironments. These cells experienced specific nutrient supply, hormonal and growth factor environments, unique cell–cell signaling, and tissue stiffness specific to the tissue in question. The new environment in vitro on a 2D substrate is foreign and hostile to primary cells derived from fresh biopsies. The new surroundings invariably force the cells to adapt to the artificial culture conditions if they are to survive in vitro. These changes could be at the gene expression level (Zaitseva, 2006) or at the epigenetic level

TABLE 5.2 Comparison of 2D and 3D Cell Culture Methods

Type of culture	2D	3D
Time of culture formation	Within minutes to a few hours	A few hours to a few days
Culture quality	High performance, reproducible, long-term culture, easy to interpret, and simplicity of culture	Worse performance and reproducibility, difficult to interpret, and difficult-to-conduct cultures
In vivo imitation	Do not mimic the natural structure of the tissue or tumor mass	Can reasonably mimic in vivo condition depending on the 3D culture system
Cell interactions	Deprived of cell–cell and cell–extracellular environment interactions, no in vivo-like microenvironment, and no "niches"	Proper interactions of cell–cell and cell–extracellular environment and environmental "niches" are created
Characteristics of cells	Changed morphology and way of divisions and loss of diverse phenotype and polarity	Preserved morphology and way of divisions, diverse phenotype, and polarity
Access to essential compounds	Unlimited access to oxygen, nutrients, metabolites and signaling molecules (in contrast to in vivo)	Variable access to oxygen, nutrients, metabolites and signaling molecules (the same as in vivo)
Molecular mechanisms	Changes in gene expression, mRNA splicing, topology, and biochemistry of cells	Expression of genes, splicing, topology, and biochemistry of cells as in vivo
Cost of maintaining a culture	Cheap, commercially available tests and media	More expensive, more time-consuming, and fewer commercially available tests

Source: Marta Kapałczyńska et al., "Comparison of 2D and 3D Cell Culture Methods" from "2D and 3D cell cultures—A Comparison of Different Types of Cancer Cell Cultures," *Archives of Medical Science*, vol. 14, no. 4. Copyright © 2018 by Termedia & Banach.

(Nestor et al., 2015; Franzen et al., 2021). With the biomedical industry gearing up to meet the need for engineered tissues and organs, newer *3D culture* techniques are being developed. Students must have an appreciation of the differences between 2D and 3D cell culture conditions and the associated advantages and disadvantages. Table 5.2 compares 2D and 3D culture methods.

Concept #6: Chemical, Microbial, and Cell–Cell Cross-Culture Contamination

Three types of contaminations are encountered in cell cultures: (a) chemical contamination (b) microbial contamination, and (c) cell-cell cross culture contamination.

Chemical Contamination

Chemical contamination occurs from reagents and vessels used for cell culture. The most common source of chemical contamination is the water used for preparing culture media, buffers, and other reagents. Glassware is another source of chemical contamination. Residual detergents from cleaned glassware, free radicals, heavy metals, and chemicals leaching out of certain types of plastic containers can harm cell cultures. The impact of these chemicals may vary with different cell lines. Chemicals used to disinfect the incubator or formaldehyde from fixed tissues when used inside the incubator have the potential to harm cell cultures if residues of the chemicals remain in vapor form for extended periods of time. Chemical contamination can be avoided or minimized to a great extent by switching to ready-to-use plasticware as culture vessels, using tissue culture grade water for preparing reagents, and avoiding the use of organic chemicals inside the culture hood and incubators.

Microbial Contamination

Microbial contamination can arise from two sources: (a) from endogenous or latent viral infections from the primary cell source and (b) accidental or adventitious contaminations during cell culture procedures. Endogenous retroviruses are stably integrated into the genome of virtually all species of animals and are genetically inherited. Some of these have the potential to produce infectious retroviruses. Dormant viruses can become activated in response to biological, immunological, and chemical agents. Spontaneous activation of retroviruses can also occur in long-term culture of cells in vitro. While viral contaminants may not be infective, they pose a serious threat in the areas of cell, tissue, and organ transplantation (for a comprehensive review, see Denner, 2017).

Microbial contaminations primarily arise from bacteria, yeast, fungus, and mycoplasma. Bacterial, yeast, and fungal contamination are readily detected because their growth can change the consistency, turbidity, and color of the culture media. Low-level growth may go undetected for some time. The incidence of bacterial, yeast, and fungal contamination can be controlled to a considerable extent with the use of antibiotic, antifungal, and antimycotic supplements in the culture medium (see Table 4.1, Chapter 4). Long-term use of antibiotics in culture can lead to antibiotic resistance. Antibiotics may also affect gene expression patterns in eukaryotic cells (Niehues et al., 2020). Therefore, careful consideration must be given to the use of antibiotics. Some labs avoid the use of antibiotics. To avoid biological contamination in those cases, extra precaution is warranted. The best recourse in the event of microbial contamination is to disinfect and discard the cultures and start fresh from frozen stocks.

Mycoplasma is different from bacteria, yeast, and fungus. It belongs to a class of bacteria called "mollicutes." These are the smallest known self-replicating bacteria (0.3 μm to 0.8 μm) and lack a cell wall. Due to their small size, *Mycoplasma* cannot be detected with regular microscopes. *Mycoplasmas* are slow-growing organisms with a long lag phase. Therefore, *Mycoplasma* contamination can go unnoticed for a long time. By the time *Mycoplasma* contamination is detected, it is highly likely to have contaminated every culture in that laboratory. They mostly grow on the outside of the eukaryotic cell membranes through a process termed "cytadherence." Some *Mycoplasma* species have been found to grow inside epithelial cells and phagocytic cells. The incidence of *Mycoplasma* contamination in cell lines ranges from about 1% in primary cells to 5% in early passage cell cultures and up to 15–35% in continuous human or animal cell lines. *M. orale*, found in the oral cavity of healthy individuals accounts for about 20 to 40% of all *Mycoplasma* infections in cell culture. Anti-*Mycoplasma* antibiotics, such as tiamulin, minocycline, ciprofloxacin, enrofloxacin, sparfloxacin, and *Mycoplasma* removal antibiotic (MRA) have been used with varying degrees of success. Long-term use of these anti-*Mycoplasma* reagents may be detrimental to eukaryotic cells (Drexler & Uphoff, 2002). A gradual slowing down of cell culture with no other "apparent" contributory factor over a period of time is indicative of *Mycoplasma* contamination. *Mycoplasma* testing kits and reagents are available. Regular testing for *Mycoplasma* should be implemented as a good laboratory practice. Any culture or reagent that tests positive for mycoplasma should be autoclaved and disposed. Autoclaving is the only reliable way to eliminate mycoplasma. One should never try to rescue contaminated cultures, unless they are rare, valuable, or irreplaceable. Work benches, biosafety cabinets and incubators should be cleaned with appropriate reagents (see Uphoff & Drexler, 2011 for detailed information).

Cell–Cell Cross-Culture Contamination

Cell–cell cross-culture contamination or *cross-culture contamination* can be defined as the unintentional contamination of one cell line by another cell line, usually by an established cell line. Two types of cross-culture contaminations can occur: interspecies and intraspecies contaminations. Interspecies contamination is relatively easy to detect based on immunological and karyotypic methods. Interspecies contamination was first reported in the early 1960s by Defendi et al. (1960) and Brand and Sylverton (1962). However, intraspecies contamination was hard to detect in the early days of cell culture due to lack of high-resolution methods.

In his seminal work entitled "Apparent HeLa Cell Contamination of Human Heteroploid Cell Lines" published in *Nature* in 1968, Stanley M. Gartler increased awareness of the dangers of sloppy handling of cell cultures and intraspecies cell–cell cross contamination. He surveyed 20 heteroploid human cell lines obtained from ATCC, research laboratories, and commercial sources, for the presence of isoforms of glucose-6-phosphate dehydrogenase (G6PD) and phosphoglucomutase (PGM). The isoforms could be distinguished by the variation in their electrophoretic mobility. G6PD has two variants (the fast type, A, A–, and the slow type, B). The fast variant (A, A–) is present exclusively in the African American population. PGM has three variants (1, 1–2, and 2) with frequencies of approximately 65%, 20%, and 15%, respectively, in both the African American and Caucasian populations. His survey revealed that all 20 cell lines expressed G6PD fast type A and PGM type 1. Even though the origins of all 20 cell lines were not known, he knew that at least 4 of the 20 cell lines were of Caucasian origin (KB, WISH, prostate, and CMP) and one cell line was from an African American female (HeLa). In his assessment, "the probability of all being G6PD A and PGM I by chance sampling is absurdly low (with values of 0·3 for A and 0·65 for PGM 1, the probability is 6×10^{-15})" (Gartler, 1968). He went to great lengths to prove that the enzyme isoforms were stable and did not spontaneously mutate in long-term cultures of established cell lines (Auersperg & Gartler, 1970). In the end, he came to the assessment that the most likely explanation for this phenomenon was the contamination from HeLa cells. He suggested that testing of cell markers should be used routinely in cell culture labs as the best guarantee against cross-culture contamination.

Immediately after Gartler's findings, a series of publications by Nelson-Rees et al. (1974, 1977, 1981) and Hay (1991) and more recent publications by Allen et al. (2016) and Korch et al. (2021) indicate the widespread nature of cross-culture contaminations. MacLeod et al. (1999) pointed to the havoc such contaminations can have on scientific research. In a survey of 252 tumor-derived cell lines from DSMZ and five other cell repositories, they concluded that widespread high levels of cross-contaminants occurred, affecting 45 cell lines supplied by 27 of 93 originators. In their analysis, the most prolific cross contaminant cell lines were HeLa, T-24, SK-HEP-1, and U-937. The authors warn that "the misidentified cell lines reported here have already been unwittingly used in several hundreds of potentially misleading reports, including use as inappropriate tumor models and subclones masquerading as independent replicates." The authors go on to state that they "believe these findings indicate a grave and chronic problem demanding radical measures, to include extra controls over cell line authentication, provenance and availability." In a survey of 483 mammalian cell culturists across 48 countries, Buehring et al. (2004) found that HeLa contaminants were used by 9% of the respondents. Only about a third of respondents tested for the identity of their cell lines. The remarkable finding was that 35% of the researchers obtained their cells from another laboratory instead of a repository. According to them, between the years of 1969 and 2004, over 220 publications in the PubMed database reported studies using cell lines contaminated with HeLa cells. In another stunning revelation, Drexler et al. (2003), in a survey of 550 leukemia cell lines, found that a fair number of cross-culture contaminations occurred with the originators of cell lines. MacLeod et al. (1999) also point to the role of cell line originators as a potential starting point for cross culture contaminations. They identify three types of contaminated cell lines:

- **virtual:** a cell line that was cross-contaminated early in development that took over the culture with no trace of the putative "new" cell type
- **misidentified:** cross-contaminated subsequent to establishment of the new cell type such that the current culture contains a mixture of the original prototype and the contaminant
- **misclassified:** unwittingly established from an unintended (often normal) cell type

All these point to the dangers of trusting a colleague with a cell line and how scientific publications using spurious cell lines can affect research outcomes, not to mention the negative impact it can have, particularly on clinical trials. These findings prompted researchers in the field to ask for proactive measures so that mishaps could be eliminated (Markovic & Markovic, 1999; Nardone, 2007). Baust et al. (2017) suggests a list of "best practices" for cell culturists.

Guidance documents stressing the need for cell line authentication prior to publication of research articles have been published (Almeida et al., 2023; Geraghty et al., 2014; Souren et al., 2022). The International Cell Line Authentication Committee (ICLAC) was established in 2012 "to make cell line misidentification more visible and to promote awareness and authentication testing as effective ways to combat it" (https://iclac.org/about-iclac/). According to the ICLAC website, "The group came together after publication of an ANSI Standard (ANSI/ATCC ASN-0002-2011), setting out the best practices for authentication testing of human cell lines. It maintains a register of cross-contaminated or otherwise misidentified cell lines and a website of resources for authentication testing." Their "Misidentified Cell Lines database" lists known false cell lines. Cellosaurus is a resource center for cell lines that provides research resource identifiers (RRIs) for cell lines (https://www.cellosaurus.org/) with the aim of potentially reducing the use of misidentified cell lines in research publications (Babic et al., 2019). To reduce the impact of misidentified cell lines, ICLAC recommends the following:

1. Check the register of known misidentified cell lines before starting work.
2. Incorporate authentication testing into everyday culture practice.
3. Report testing as an essential part of publications and grant applications.

Methods For Cell Line Identification

Cell lines can be identified using a variety of techniques:

- isoenzyme analysis (e.g., G6PD and PGM)
- karyotyping (more useful to identify interspecies contamination)
- human lymphocyte antigen (HLA) typing
- amplified fragment length polymorphisms (AFLP) analysis
- single nucleotide polymorphism (SNP) analysis
- DNA bar coding
- short tandem repeat (STR) profiling

Table 5.3 presents the relative advantages and applications of commonly used cell identification methods. Cell authentication resources are available on the National Institute's website (https://www.ncbi.nlm.nih.gov/biosample/docs/authenticate/). *STR profiling is the preferred method and is used widely for the following reasons*:

- high discriminatory power
- established testing infrastructure
- cost-effectiveness
- effective for degraded DNA samples
- comparability of STR profiling data from various platforms
- ability to detect human DNA mixtures

TABLE 5.3 SNP, STR, and DNA Barcode Technologies as Standard Methods for Assessing the Identity of Cell Lines From Different Species

Species	Assays	Consensus standard method	Commercially available kit	Commercial service
Human	STR	ASN-0002	Yes	Yes
	SNP	No	Yes	Yes
Mouse	STR	No	No	Yes
	SNP	No	Yes	Yes
African green monkey	STR	No	No	No
Chinese hamster ovary	STR	No	No	No
Rat	STR	No	No	No
Species-level identification	CO1 DNA barcode	ASN-0003	Yes	Yes
	Species-specific primers	No	No	Yes

Adapted from Jamie L Almeida, Kenneth D Cole and Anne L Plant, "SNP, STR, and DNA Barcode Technologies" from "Standards for Cell Line Authentication and Beyond," *PLoS Biology*, vol, 14, no. 6, 2016.

Variation Within Cell Lines

A less appreciated problem with cell lines is the possibility of variation within a pure cell line over extended periods of in vitro culturing. Such variations occur due to a phenomenon called "genetic drift" or "allelic drift" or by mutations such as deletions, duplications, insertions, inversions, SNPs, and altered gene expression patterns. Most cancer cell lines, by their very nature, are bound to carry mutations and may undergo rapid genetic diversification as a result of positive clonal selection. Culture conditions and frequency of passaging may have greater effect on genetic drift (Ben-David et al., 2018). One of the earliest incidences of genetic drift in established cell lines was reported by Baker et al. (1979) in HeLa cells. They found that a new strain of HeLa cells derived from the original HeLa line differed in its sensitivity to ethyl methane sulfonate. Similarly, genetic drifts in the U-251 glioblastoma cell line (Torsvik et al., 2014), lymphoblastoid cell lines (Joesch-Cohen et al., 2017), and DNA methylation changes in long-term culture of mesenchymal stem cells (Franzen et al., 2021) have been reported. Certain cell lines may be more prone to extensive clonotypic heterogeneity compared to other cell lines. For example, Parson et al. (2005) reported that cell lines U-937 and K-562 exhibited a high degree of stability and clonotypic homogeneity after long-term culture, whereas CCRF-CEM and Jurkat cells revealed extensive clonotypic heterogeneity, with subclones differing in up to eight STR loci from the parental culture.

Chapter Takeaways

- PDL reflects the "true age" of cells, not the passage number. PDL specifically applies to primary cells and indicates how close these cells are to Hayflick limit and senescence.
- Primary cells have a finite lifespan. The physiology of cells at PDL 40 is likely to be vastly different from PDL 20. Research involving primary cells should always consider using cells within a narrow range of PDL to obtain consistent results. It is a good practice to freeze cells at low passage/PDL so that one can go back to "young" cells for consistency within that experiment.
- The "true age" of cells derived from a fetus, a 10-year-old, and a 40-year-old will exhibit different physiologies due to their age differences. Cells from older individuals reach the Hayflick limit faster than cells from young individuals.
- The age of cells should be a major consideration when using cells for cellular therapies and organ engineering.
- Cell behavior and gene expression patterns in 2D and 3D culture can vary significantly.
- It takes time for cells to adapt when switched from a 2D culture to a 3D culture. The growth rate and morphology will change.
- Good laboratory practices must be followed to prevent chemical and microbial contamination. Constant monitoring should be practiced to avoid or minimize microbial contamination. Any contaminated cultures should be treated with 10% bleach and discarded immediately.
- Cell–cell cross-culture contamination is a bane of the cell culture community. Precautions should be taken to ensure that uncontaminated cell lines are used for experimentation. Best practices to monitor the purity of cell lines should be established in every lab.
- Pure cell lines can undergo genetic drift in long-term cultures. This can happen independently in cell culture labs. Therefore, results with the same cell line can differ significantly between different labs.

References

Allen, M., Bjerke, M., Edlund, H., Nelander, S., & Westermark, B. (2016). Origin of the U87MG glioma cell line: Good news and bad news. *Sci Transl Med.*, *8*(354), 354re3. https://www.doi.org/10.1126/scitranslmed.aaf6853. PMID: 27582061.

Almeida, J. L., Cole, K. D., & Plant, A. L. (2016). Standards for cell line authentication and beyond. *PLoS Biol.*, *14*(6), e1002476. https://www.doi.org/10.1371/journal.pbio.1002476. PMID: 27300367; PMCID: PMC4907466.

Almeida, J. L., & Korch, C. T. (2023). Authentication of human and mouse cell lines by short tandem repeat (STR) DNA genotype analysis. In S. Markossian, A. Grossman, & K. Brimacombe (Eds.), *Assay guidance manual*. Eli Lilly & Company and the National Center for Advancing Translational Sciences. https://www.ncbi.nlm.nih.gov/books/NBK144066/

Auersperg, N., & Gartler, S. M. (1970). Isoenzyme stability in human heteroploid cell lines. *Experimental Cell Research*, *61*(2), 465–7. https://www.doi.org/10.1016/0014-4827(70)90474-x. PMID: 5459846.

Babic, Z., Capes-Davis, A., Martone, M. E., Bairoch, A., Ozyurt, I. B., Gillespie, T. H., & Bandrowski, A. E. (2019). Incidences of problematic cell lines are lower in papers that use RRIDs to identify cell lines. *Elife*, *8*, e41676. https://www.doi.org/10.7554/eLife.41676. PMID: 30693867; PMCID: PMC6351100.

Baker, R. M., Van Voorhis, W. C., & Spencer, L. A. (1979). HeLa cell variants that differ in sensitivity to monofunctional alkylating agents, with independence of cytotoxic and mutagenic responses. *Proceedings of the National Academy of Sciences U S A*, *76*(10), 5249–53. https://www.doi.org/v10.1073/pnas.76.10.5249. PMID: 291942; PMCID: PMC413118.

Bashor, C. J., Hilton, I. B., Bandukwala, H., Smith, D. M., & Veiseh, O. (2022). Engineering the next generation of cell-based therapeutics. *Nature Reviews Drug Discovery*, *21*(9), 655–675. https://www.doi.org/10.1038/s41573-022-00476-6. PMID: 35637318; PMCID: PMC9149674.

Baust, J. M., Buehring, G. C., Campbell, L., Elmore, E., Harbell, J. W., Nims, R. W., Price, P., Reid, Y. A., & Simione, F. (2017). Best practices in cell culture: An overview. In *Vitro Cellular & Developmental Biology—Animal*, *53*(8), 669–672. https://www.doi.org/10.1007/s11626-017-0177-7. PMID: 28808859.

Brand, K. G., & Syverton, J. T. (1962). Results of species-specific hemagglutination tests on "transformed," nontransformed, and primary cell cultures. *Journal of the National Cancer Institute*, *28*, 147–57. PMID: 13872458.

Ben-David, U., Siranosian, B., Ha, G., Tang, H., Oren, Y., Hinohara, K., Strathdee, C. A., Dempster, J., Lyons, N. J., Burns, R., Nag, A., Kugener, G., Cimini, B., Tsvetkov, P., Maruvka, Y. E., O'Rourke, R., Garrity, A., Tubelli, A. A., Bandopadhayay, P., Golub, T. R. (2018). Genetic and transcriptional evolution alters cancer cell line drug response. *Nature*, *560*(7718), 325–330. https://www.doi.org/10.1038/s41586-018-0409-3. PMID: 30089904; PMCID: PMC6522222.

Buehring, G. C., Eby, E. A., & Eby, M. J. (2004). Cell line cross-contamination: How aware are Mammalian cell culturists of the problem and how to monitor it? In *Vitro Cellular & Developmental Biology—Animal*, *40*(7), 2115. https://www.doi.org/10.1290/1543-706X(2004)40<211:CLCHAA>2.0.CO;2. PMID: 15638703.

Carrel, A. (1912). On the permanent life of tissues outside of the organism. *Journal of Experimental Medicine*, *15*(5), 516–28. https://www.doi.org/10.1084/jem.15.5.516. PMID: 19867545; PMCID: PMC2124948.

Denner, J. (2017). The porcine virome and xenotransplantation. *Virology Journal*, *14*(1), 171. https://www.doi.org/10.1186/s12985-017-0836-z. PMID: 28874166; PMCID: PMC5585927.

Defendi, V., Billingham, R. E., Silvers, W. K., & Moorhead, P. (1960). Immunological and karyological criteria for identification of cell lines. *Journal of the National Cancer Institute*, *25*, 359–85. PMID: 13815376.

Drexler, H. G., & Uphoff, C. C. (2002). Mycoplasma contamination of cell cultures: Incidence, sources, effects, detection, elimination, prevention. *Cytotechnology*, *39*(2), 75–90. https://www.doi.org/10.1023/A:1022913015916. PMID: 19003295; PMCID: PMC3463982.

Drexler, H. G., Dirks, W. G., Matsuo, Y., & MacLeod, R. A. (2003). False leukemia-lymphoma cell lines: An update on over 500 cell lines. *Leukemia*, *17*(2), 416–26. https://www.doi.org/10.1038/sj.leu.2402799. PMID: 12592342.

Durkin, M. E., Qian, X., Popescu, N. C., & Lowy, D. R. (2013). Isolation of mouse embryo fibroblasts. *Bio Protocol.*, *3*(18), e908. https://www.doi.org/10.21769/bioprotoc.908. PMID: 27376106; PMCID: PMC4928858.

Ebeling, A. H. (1922). A ten year old strain of fibroblasts. *Journal of Experimental Medicine*, *35*(6), 755–9. https://www.doi.org/10.1084/jem.35.6.755. PMID: 19868644; PMCID: PMC2128318.

Franzen, J., Georgomanolis, T., Selich, A., Kuo, C. C., Stöger, R., Brant, L., Mulabdić, M. S., Fernandez-Rebollo, E., Grezella, C., Ostrowska, A., Begemann, M., Nikolić, M., Rath, B., Ho, A. D., Rothe, M., Schambach, A., Papantonis, A., & Wagner, W. (2021). DNA methylation changes during long-term in vitro cell culture are caused by epigenetic drift. *Communications Biology—Nature*, *4*(1), 598. https://www.doi.org/10.1038/s42003-021-02116-y. PMID: 34011964; PMCID: PMC8134454.

Gartler, S. (1968). Apparent HeLa cell contamination of human heteroploid cell lines. *Nature*, *217*, 750–751. https://doi.org/10.1038/217750a0

Geraghty, R. J., Capes-Davis, A., Davis, J. M., Downward, J., Freshney, R. I., Knezevic, I., Lovell-Badge, R., Masters, J. R., Meredith, J., Stacey, G. N., Thraves, P., & Vias, M. (2014). Cancer Research UK: Guidelines for the use of cell lines in biomedical research. *British Journal of Cancer*, *111*(6), 1021–46. https://www.doi.org/10.1038/bjc.2014.166. PMID: 25117809; PMCID: PMC4453835.

Hay, R. J. (1991). Operator-induced contamination in cell culture systems. *Developments in biological standardization.*, *75*, 193–204. PMID: 1794620.

Hayflick, L., & Moorhead, P. S. (1961). The serial cultivation of human diploid cell strains. *Experimental Cell Research*, *25*, 585621. https://www.doi.org/10.1016/0014-4827(61)90192-6. PMID: 13905658.

Hayflick, L. (1965). The limited in vitro lifetime of human diploid cell strains. *Experimental Cell Research.*, *37*, 614–36. https://www.doi.org/10.1016/0014-4827(65)90211-9. PMID: 14315085.

Hayflick, L. (1998). A brief history of the mortality and immortality of cultured cells. *The Keio Journal of Medicine*, *47*(3), 174–82. https://www.doi.org/10.2302/kjm.47.174. PMID: 9785764.

Joesch-Cohen, L. M., & Glusman, G. (2017). Differences between the genomes of lymphoblastoid cell lines and blood-derived samples. *Journal of Advances In Genomics and Genetics*, *7*:1–9. https://www.doi.org/10.2147/AGG.S128824. PMID: 28736497; PMCID: PMC5520659.

Kapałczyńska, M., Kolenda, T., Przybyła, W., Zajączkowska, M., Teresiak, A., Filas, V., Ibbs, M., Bliźniak, R., Łuczewski, Ł., & Lamperska, K. (2018). 2D and 3D cell cultures: A comparison of different types of cancer cell cultures. *Archives of Medical Science*, *14*(4), 910–919. https://www.doi.org/10.5114/aoms.2016.63743. PMID: 30002710; PMCID: PMC6040128.

Khorraminejad-Shirazi, M., Dorvash, M., Estedlal, A., Hoveidaei, A. H., Mazloomrezaei, M., & Mosaddeghi, P. (2019). Aging: A cell source limiting factor in tissue engineering. *World Journal of Stem Cells, 11*(10), 787–802. https://www.doi.org/10.4252/wjsc.v11.i10.787. PMID: 31692986; PMCID: PMC6828594.

Korch, C. T., & Capes-Davis A. (2021). The extensive and expensive impacts of HEp-2 [HeLa], intestine 407 [HeLa], and other false cell lines in journal publications. *SLAS Discovery, 26*(10), 1268–1279. https://www.doi.org/10.1177/24725552211051963. PMID: 34697958.

MacLeod, R. A., Dirks, W. G., Matsuo, Y., Kaufmann, M., Milch, H., & Drexler, H. G. (1999). Widespread intraspecies cross-contamination of human tumor cell lines arising at source. *International Journal of Cancer, 83*(4), 555–63. https://www.doi.org/10.1002/(sici)1097-0215(19991112)83:4<555::aid-ijc19>3.0.co;2-2. PMID: 10508494.

Markovic, O., & Markovic, N. (1998). Cell cross-contamination in cell cultures: The silent and neglected danger. In *Vitro Cellular & Developmental Biology—Animal, 34*(1), 1–8. https://www.doi.org/10.1007/s11626-998-0040-y. PMID: 9542623.

Nardone, R. M. (2007). Eradication of cross-contaminated cell lines: A call for action. *Cell Biology and Toxicology, 23*(6), 367–72. https://www.doi.org/10.1007/s10565-007-9019-9. PMID: 17522957.

Nejaddehbashi, F., Bayati, V., Mashali, L., Hashemitabar, M., Abbaspour, M., Moghimipour, E., & Orazizadeh, M. (2019). Isolating human dermal fibroblasts using serial explant culture. *Stem Cell Investigation, 6*, 23. https://www.doi.org/10.21037/sci.2019.08.05. PMID: 31559310; PMCID: PMC6737403.

Nelson-Rees, W. A., Flandermeyer, R. R., & Hawthorne, P. K. (1974). Banded marker chromosomes as indicators of intraspecies cellular contamination. *Science, 184*(4141), 1093–6. https://www.doi.org/10.1126/science.184.4141.1093. PMID: 4469665.

Nelson-Rees, W. A., & Flandermeyer, R. R. (1977). Inter- and intraspecies contamination of human breast tumor cell lines HBC and BrCa5 and other cell cultures. *Science, 195*(4284), 1343–4. https://www.doi.org/10.1126/science.557237. PMID: 557237.

Nelson-Rees, W. A., Hunter, L., Darlington, G. J., & O'Brien, S. J. (1980). Characteristics of HeLa strains: Permanent vs. variable features. *Cytogenetics and Cell Genetics, 27*(4), 216–31. https://www.doi.org/10.1159/000131490. PMID: 7002488.

Nelson-Rees, W. A., Daniels, D. W., & Flandermeyer, R. R. (1981). Cross-contamination of cells in culture. *Science, 212*(4493), 446–52. https://www.doi.org/10.1126/science.6451928. PMID: 6451928.

Nestor, C. E., Ottaviano, R., Reinhardt, D., Cruickshanks, H. A., Mjoseng, H. K., McPherson, R. C., Lentini, A., Thomson, J. P., Dunican, D. S., Pennings, S., Anderton, S. M., Benson, M., & Meehan, R. R. (2015). Rapid reprogramming of epigenetic and transcriptional profiles in mammalian culture systems. *Genome Biology, 16*(1), 11. https://www.doi.org/10.1186/s13059-014-0576-y. PMID: 25648825; PMCID: PMC4334405.

Niehues, H., Jansen, P. A. M., Rodijk-Olthuis, D., Rikken, G., Smits, J. P. H., Schalkwijk, J., Zeeuwen, P. L. J. M., & van den Bogaard, E. H. J. (2020). Know your enemy: Unexpected, pervasive, and persistent viral and bacterial contamination of primary cell cultures. *Experimental Dermatology, 29*(7), 672–676. https://www.doi.org/10.1111/exd.14126. PMID: 32506526; PMCID: PMC7496648.

Ohmine, S., Squillace, K. A., Hartjes, K. A., Deeds, M. C., Armstrong, A. S., Thatava, T., Sakuma, T., Terzic, A., Kudva, Y., & Ikeda, Y. (2012). Reprogrammed keratinocytes from elderly type 2 diabetes patients suppress senescence genes to acquire induced pluripotency. *Aging, 4*(1), 60–73. https://www.doi.org/10.18632/aging.100428. PMID: 22308265; PMCID: PMC3292906.

Parson, W., Kirchebner, R., Mühlmann, R., Renner, K., Kofler, A., Schmidt, S., & Kofler, R. (2005). Cancer cell line identification by short tandem repeat profiling: Power and limitations. *The FASEB Journal, 19*(3), 434–6. https://www.doi.org/10.1096/fj.04-3062fje. PMID: 15637111.

Richter, M., Piwocka, O., Musielak, M., Piotrowski, I., Suchorska, W. M., & Trzeciak, T. (2021). From donor to the lab: A fascinating journey of primary cell lines. *Frontiers in Cell and Developmental Biology, 9*, 711381. https://www.doi.org/10.3389/fcell.2021.711381. PMID: 34395440; PMCID: PMC8356673.

Shannon, J. L., Kirchner, S. J., & Zhang, J. Y. (2022). Human skin explant preparation and culture. *Bio-protocol Journal*, 12(18), e4514. https://www.doi.org/10.21769/BioProtoc.4514. PMID: 36248607; PMCID: PMC9516224.

Souren, N. Y., Fusenig, N. E., Heck, S., Dirks, W. G., Capes-Davis, A., Bianchini, F., & Plass, C. (2022). Cell line authentication: A necessity for reproducible biomedical research. *The EMBO Journal, 41*(14), e111307. https://www.doi.org/10.15252/embj.2022111307. PMID: 35758134; PMCID: PMC9289526.

Torsvik, A., Stieber, D., Enger, P. Ø., Golebiewska, A., Molven, A., Svendsen, A., Westermark, B., Niclou, S. P., Olsen, T. K., Chekenya Enger, M., & Bjerkvig R. (2014). U-251 revisited: Genetic drift and phenotypic consequences of long-term cultures of glioblastoma cells. *Cancer Medicine, 3*(4), 812–24. https://www.doi.org/10.1002/cam4.219. PMID: 24810477; PMCID: PMC4303149.

Uphoff, C. C., & Drexler, H. G. (2011). Elimination of mycoplasmas from infected cell lines using antibiotics. *Methods in Molecular Biology, 731*, 105–14. https://www.doi.org/10.1007/978-1-61779-080-5_9. PMID: 21516401.

Verma, A., Verma, M., & Singh, A. (2020). Animal tissue culture principles and applications. *Animal Biotechnology*, 269–93. https://www.doi.org/10.1016/B978-0-12-811710-1.00012-4. PMCID: PMC7325846.

Wen, Y., Wani, P., Zhou, L., Baer, T., Phadnis, S. M., Reijo Pera, R. A., & Chen, B. (2013). Reprogramming of fibroblasts from older women with pelvic floor disorders alters cellular behavior associated with donor age. *Stem Cells Translational Medicine*, 2(2), 118–28. https://www.doi.org/10.5966/sctm.2012-0092. PMID: 23341439; PMCID: PMC3659753.

Witkowski, J. A. (1980). Dr. Carrel's immortal cells. *Medical history*, 24(2), 129–42. https://www.doi.org/10.1017/s0025727300040126. PMID: 6990125; PMCID: PMC1082700.

Zaitseva, M., Vollenhoven, B. J., & Rogers, P. A. (2006). In vitro culture significantly alters gene expression profiles and reduces differences between myometrial and fibroid smooth muscle cells. *Molecular Human Reproduction*, 12(3), 187–207. https://www.doi.org/10.1093/molehr/gal018. PMID: 16524927.

Credit

UNIT II

Detailed Experimental Protocols

Basic Protocols

Protocol for Routine Subculturing and Passaging of Mammalian Cells

---

Objectives

- ✓ Learn routine subculturing of mammalian cells using mouse NIH/3T3 cells as a model cell line.
- ✓ The first 2 weeks of subculture procedure will be based on split ratios. After the first 2 weeks, you will determine the cell count and seed specific cell numbers during the rest of the term as described in the "Cell counting protocol".

Procedure

1. Wear the necessary Personal Protective Equipment (gloves, safety goggles, lab coat). Sterilize the gloves by spraying 70% isopropyl alcohol.
2. Switch on the lights and air circulation for the culture hood. Open the hood sash to the optimal height as indicated on the hood.
3. Spray the surface and grill area of the culture hood with 70% isopropanol. Wipe it clean using a paper towel, starting from inside to the outside of the hood.
4. If you are using a vacuum suction set up to aspirate liquid, spray 70% isopropanol into the suction tube with the vacuum pump running. Spray outside the tube and wipe it clean.
5. Take the culture dish out of the incubator and check the color and consistency of the culture medium. Based on the degree of cell growth, the media will be red, slightly pink, or yellow in color. Cloudy media indicates possible contamination of the culture.
6. **<u>Before bringing the culture plate into the hood, observe it under the microscope</u>** to check for (1) the health of cells, (2) degree of cell confluency, and (3) absence of contamination.
7. After microscopic observation, bring the plate inside the hood.

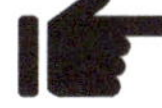

NOTE: If the culture looks cloudy and contaminated, do not bring the plate inside the culture hood. Take the culture plate to the sink and add 10% bleach. Close the lid and leave the plate in the sink overnight. After 12–24 hr of bleach treatment, discard the contents in the sink and dispose the plate in the biohazard waste container.

---

8. Take a new sterile 15 ml conical centrifuge tube. Mark the name of the cell line and other information on the tube, as necessary.
9. Attach a sterile glass Pasteur pipette to the tube attached to the vacuum pump. Carefully aspirate the medium from the culture plate. Tilting the plate to one side makes aspiration easy and efficient.
10. Using a serological pipette, gently add 5 ml of **DPBS without Ca^{++}/Mg^{++} [DPBS(-)]** along the side of the plate. Allow the DPBS(-) to wash over the surface of the plate by gently tilting the plate several times.
11. Attach a new sterile Pasteur pipette to the tube attached to the vacuum suction system. Tilt the plate to one side so that the liquid pools at the bottom. Carefully aspirate DPBS(-).
12. Using a serological pipette, gently add 3 ml of 0.25% Trypsin-EDTA solution along the side of the plate. Close the lid.
13. Transfer the plate to a 37°C incubator or a slide warmer and incubate for 5–10 min.

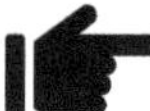

Normally, plates are incubated inside a cell culture incubator. The use of the slide warmer is a modification for this lab course to avoid depletion of CO_2 from the CO_2 tank attached to the incubator. A regular incubator without CO_2 supply may be substituted.

---

14. After incubation, check the cells under a microscope to check for the degree of trypsinization. The cells should look rounded, detached, and floating. If they look rounded, the plate is ready for further processing. Bring the plate into the hood.
15. Using a fresh serological pipette, add 7 ml **complete medium** to the plate. The FBS in the complete medium will help neutralize the proteolytic activity of trypsin. **The total volume of liquid in the plate is 10 ml (3 ml trypsin + 7 ml complete medium).**
16. Using the same serological pipette, disperse cells by repeated pipetting. **Avoid air bubbles.**
17. Transfer cell suspension to the sterile 15 ml conical tube. Repeat pipetting in the tube to break up any remaining cell clumps.

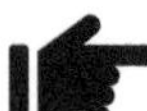

NOTE: If you plan to do a cell count, you can use a sample of cell suspension at this point.

---

18. Do a quality check on the plate. Check the plate under the microscope to ensure that there are minimal residual cells left on the plate.
19. Place the 15 ml tube containing cells in the centrifuge with the writing patch facing out. Place a balancing tube containing water of same volume or another student's cell suspension in the holder opposite your sample. Spin the tubes at **200–250 G** for 7–10 min. After centrifugation, look for the cell pellet at the bottom of the tube below the writing patch.
20. Bring the 15 ml tube into the hood. Using a sterile Pasteur pipette attached to the vacuum pump, carefully aspirate the supernatant leaving the pellet intact with less than 0.5 ml fluid in the tube.

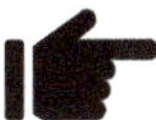

Be careful NOT to aspirate the cell pellet. To achieve this, aspirate the fluid from the top and go down with the meniscus.

21. Determine the desired split ratio. For example, if you are planning a 1:5 split, resuspend the cell pellet in 5 ml complete medium. Add 1 ml of this cell suspension to 9 ml fresh complete medium in a new culture plate. To do this, first add 9 ml of fresh complete medium to the new culture plate. Add 1 ml cell suspension to the 9 ml medium (**total volume 10 ml**). See example in the table below.

Split ratio	Pellet resuspension volume (ml)	Volume of fresh medium in 100 mm plate (ml)	Cell suspension for plating (ml)	Total volume (ml)
1:3	3	9	1	10
1:4	4	9	1	10
1:5	5	9	1	10
1:5	10	8	2	10
1:10	10	9	1	10
1:10	5	9.5	0.5	10
1:20	10	9.5	0.5	10
1:20	5	9.75	0.25	10

22. **Check the cells under a microscope.** Cells that have settled to the bottom of the plate will remain in sharp focus, while cells that are still in suspension can be observed at different focal planes and slowly coming into sharp focus as they settle to the bottom. Transfer the plate to the incubator for continued incubation for the desired duration.
23. Using vacuum suction, aspirate the remainder of the cell suspension in the 15 ml tube. Discard the used plates and tubes in the biohazard bin, clean the hood and the vacuum suction tube, and close the hood.

SUPPLY LIST—This list is for guidance only. Equivalent products may be used based on lab preferences.

Item	Vendor	Catalog #
NIH/3T3 cells	ATCC	CRL-1658
100mm × 20mm Tissue Culture Treated Dishes w/Grip Ring	Chemglass	CLS-1805-152
DMEM media (w/4.5 g/L glucose, and sodium pyruvate, no L-glutamine)	VWR	45000-316
Fetal bovine serum	Your choice	
Glutamax supplement (100×)	Thermo Fisher	35050061
Penicillin : Streptomycin solution 100×, Corning	VWR	45000-652
DPBS(-)	VWR	45000-434
4-Chip Disposable Hemocytometer, 4 chambers per chip	VWR	102966-632
Double Neubauer Chamber with 2 coverglass	VWR	102094-780

NOTE:

1. The supply list provided here is for guidance only. Equivalent products may be used based on the preferences in each lab.
2. Some labs may prefer using only 0.1% Trypsin-EDTA. In the context of a teaching lab, 0.25% Trypsin-EDTA ensures efficient trypsinization.
3. The CellTreat brand of culture plates from Chemglass has a grip ring for convenient handling of plates for students new to cell culture.

Cell Counting Protocol

What should you expect to learn in this lab?

1. What is a hemocytometer?
2. Factors affecting cell count.
3. Cell counting procedure.

Determination of Cell Count

In this lab, you will determine cell count using the C-Chip disposable hemocytometer. For most experiments, it is important to use a consistent **plating density.** In this procedure, cells are trypsinized and resuspended in a specific volume. You will use a small volume of this cell suspension after trypsinization and neutralization to perform cell count using a hemocytometer. The cell suspension is added through the loading area in the hemocytometer to allow filling the counting chamber by capillary action. **It is important not to force-fill the counting chamber.** The counting area in the C-chip disposable hemocytometer holds 6 µl for the four-chamber slides. The counting area in the Neubauer hemocytometer holds 10 µl for the counting area (see images below).

Some important pointers to bear in mind:

- **Proper mixing is essential for accurate cell count.** Close the cap of the tube containing the cell suspension and mix the contents by inverting the tube a few times before drawing a sample for cell counting.
- **Appropriate concentration:** To obtain a good cell count, the concentration of the cells in the counting area should not be too low or too high. A total count between 50 and 200 in the four corner chambers combined is a desirable number. Fewer cells per square can result in a higher error rate. If this happens, centrifuge the sample again and resuspend the pellet in a smaller volume. If the cell concentration is too high, dilute a small volume of cell suspension in basal media or DPBS as deemed necessary (for e.g., a dilution of 1:2, 1:3, 1:5 etc.). **Never use water to dilute cells as this will cause osmotic shock and cell rupture.** When diluting the suspension, the dilution factor must be considered when calculating the final concentration.

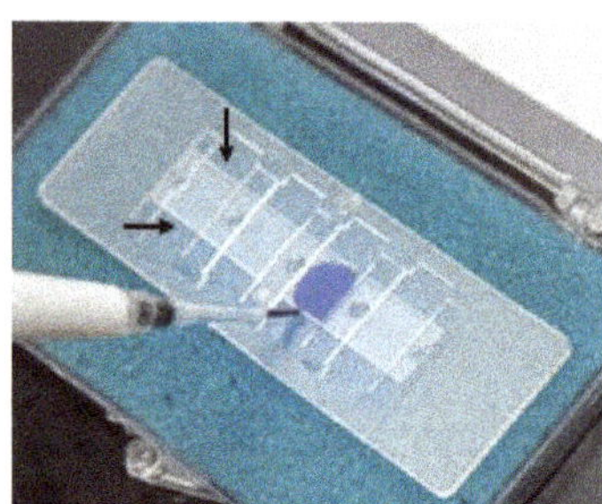
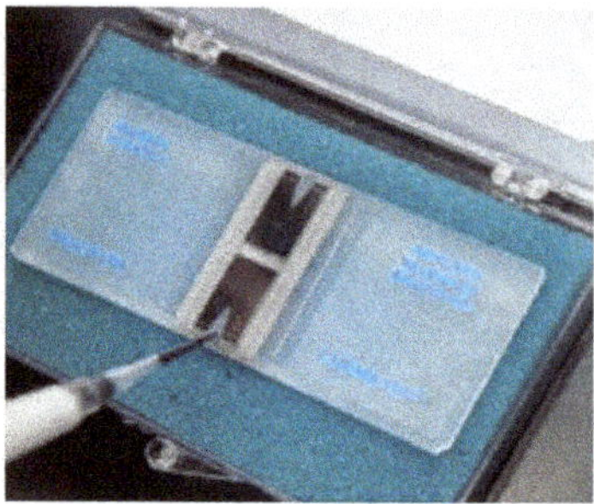

FIGURE BP 2.1 C-Chip disposable hemocytometer (left) and Neubauer hemocytometer (right). Note the four chambers in the C-chip hemocytometer. It can be loaded from either side (arrows).

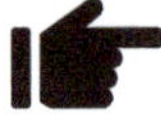

TIP: It is important **NOT** to underload or overload the chamber. Care should be taken to fill the chamber without air bubbles. It is also important to perform counting soon after loading to prevent the sample from drying.

Figures BP 2.2a and BP 2.2b illustrates how to count and which cells to count using a hemocytometer.

Start counting from the top left corner square within each large corner square and proceed in a zigzag fashion, counting all 16 small squares (Figure BP 2.2a). Include cells on the left and top edges and exclude cells on the right and bottom edges (Figure BP 2.2b).

Calculating cell count

Step 1—Averaging: For large eukaryotic cells you will count cells in the four large corner squares. Determine the average cell number per corner square.

Step 2—Computing the volume: It is necessary to determine the volume represented by the corner square. The area of the square (1 mm × 1 mm) must be multiplied by the height of the sample (0.1 mm). The total volume of one corner square V = 1 mm × 1 mm × 0.1 mm = 0.1 mm^3 (100 nl = 1/10,000 ml).

Step 3—Calculating the number of cells in 1 ml: Multiply the average number of cells per large corner square by a factor of 10,000 to obtain **cell numbers per ml**.

Step 4—Correcting for dilution: If you added trypan blue stain to the suspension (see note below) or if the sample was diluted before counting, then the dilution factor must be taken into consideration for calculating cell number.

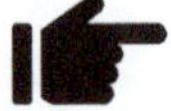

Cell count/ml of suspension = Average count per square × dilution factor × 10,000

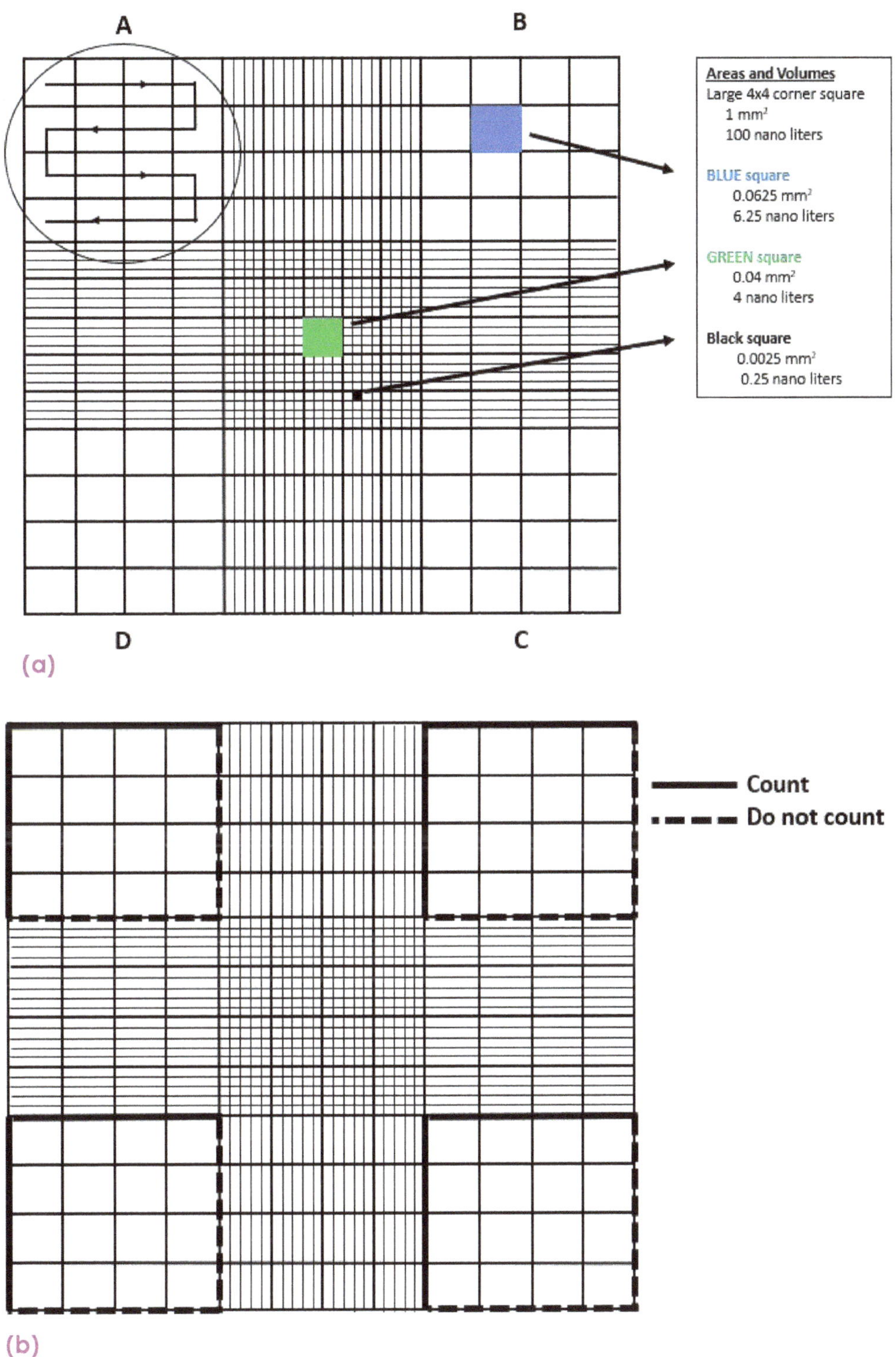

FIGURE BP 2.2 Cell Counting Protocol

Step 5—Determine total cell count: This can be done by multiplying the above number (from step 4) by the **total volume** of cell suspension from which the sample was drawn for counting (5 ml in your case).

Useful tip:

Typically, after centrifugation, cell pellets are resuspended at multiples of million cells per ml of medium (e.g., 0.25, 0.5, 1, or 2 million cells/ml). In this course, it is suggested that the cells be resuspended at 1×10^6 cells per milliliter. If you determine the total number to be 3.3 million cells, resuspend cells in 3.3 ml media for 1 million cells per ml. Resuspending cells at 1×10^6 cells per ml yields 1,000 cells per microliter. This makes it convenient to calculate the volume of cell suspension to be seeded. For example, to seed 250,000 cells per well, seed 250 µl of the above cell suspension. Similarly, use 100 µl, 200 µl, 500 µl, and 1000 µl to seed 100,000, 200,000, 500,000, and 1 million cells, respectively.

SUPPLY LIST—This list is for guidance only. Equivalent products may be used based on lab preferences.

Item	Vendor	Cat #
4-Chip Disposable Hemocytometer, four chambers per chip	VWR	102966-632
Double Neubauer Chamber with two Cover glass	VWR	102094-780
Cell counting clicker	Any brand	

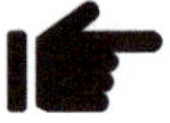

NOTE: If one needs to determine cell viability, trypan blue staining may be performed. Resuspend the cell pellets in DPBS (the presence of serum can yield misleading results). Mix equal volumes of 0.4% Trypan blue stock and cell suspension. After 3 min of incubation, count the cells as described above. Counting should be performed within 3–5 min after trypan blue incubation. Dead cells, by virtue of compromised cell membranes, will stain blue. Count unstained cells (viable) and stained cells (dead). Determine percent viability. Multiply the yield by a factor of 2 to account for the dilution factor.

Live and Dead Staining of Cells

What should you expect to learn in this lab?

1. Purpose of live/dead staining of cells.
2. Understand the various dyes that can differentiate live and dead cells.
3. Application of differentiating live and dead cells.

Materials Provided

1. Required PPE (lab coat, gloves, safety goggles)
2. One 12-well plate per student, containing mouse NIH/3T3 cells, seeded at a density of about 50,000 cells per well the day prior to the lab
3. DMEM complete medium
4. Ice-cold methanol
5. Hoechst 33342 stock—0.5 μg/ml in DPBS(+) and culture media
6. DAPI stock—200 ng/ml in DPBS(+) and culture media
7. Propidium iodide stock—0.2 μg/ml in DPBS(+) and culture media

Treat the cells as per the template and the protocol below. Observe cells under a fluorescent microscope after staining and image the cells. Note down your observations.

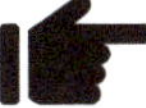

NOTE: Do not let the cells dry out during the procedure.

	Dead stain Fix cells in methanol	Live stain No methanol fixation	No stain control		
Treatment	Rinse with DPBS **with** Ca++/ Mg++ Fix with methanol	None	None		
	1	2	3	4	**Treatment**
A				Blank	Hoechst stain
B				Blank	DAPI stain
C				Blank	Propidium iodide stain
Staining	Add stain in DPBS (+)	Add stain in complete media	No stain control		

Procedure

Be gentle when you add reagents and aspirate fluid from the wells. Shear forces can lift the cells off the plate.

1. Aspirate media from wells in column 1 using a P-1000 pipette. Leave columns 2 and 3 as it is.
2. To column 1, add 1 ml DPBS (+), rinse by gentle swirling. Aspirate and discard DPBS (+).
3. Repeat DPBS (+) rinse one more time. Aspirate and discard.

   USE EYE PROTECTION WHILE HANDLING METHANOL FIXATIVE
4. Add 1 ml ice-cold methanol to the three wells in column 1.
5. Let it stand for 10 minutes at room temperature. Methanol fixes and permeabilizes the cells.
6. After the incubation, aspirate, and discard methanol from wells in column 1.
7. Add 1 ml DPBS (+) to all wells in column 1, rinse, and discard. Repeat DPBS (+) rinse one more time.
8. Aspirate **DPBS from all wells in column 1** and **media from all wells in column 2.**
9. To wells in column 1, add 1 ml stain prepared in DPBS(+) as as indicated in the **Treatment** column in the figure above.
10. To wells in column 2, add 1 ml stain prepared in complete media as as indicated in the **Treatment** column in the figure above.
11. Cover the plates with silver foil and let it incubate in the incubator for 15–20 min.
12. After the incubation period, aspirate the staining solution from all wells.
13. Rinse all wells twice with 1 ml DPBS(+).
14. Add 1 ml DPBS(+) without stain to wells in column 1 and complete media without stain to all wells in columns 2 and 3.
15. Image cells using phase contrast and fluorescence microscopy. Hoechst and DAPI can be detected using the blue filter. Propidium iodide can be detected using the red filter.
16. Determine the ability of each dye to stain live and dead cells.

Results Review

1. What is the pattern of staining in the methanol-fixed (dead) cells with Hoechst, DAPI, and propidium iodide stains?
2. What is the pattern of staining in unfixed cells (live, column 2) with Hoechst, DAPI, and propidium iodide stains?
3. Which cells are stained with Hoechst stain (live/dead)?
4. Which cells are stained with DAPI stain (live/dead)?
5. Which cells are stained with propidium iodide stain (live/dead)?
6. If you want to stain both live and dead cells in a culture, what dye combination would you choose to distinguish live and dead cells?

SUPPLY LIST—This list is for guidance only. Equivalent products may be used based on lab preferences.

Item	Vendor	Catalog #
NIH/3T3 cells	ATCC	CRL-1658
DMEM media (w/4.5 g/L glucose, and sodium pyruvate, no L-glutamine)	VWR	45000-316
Fetal bovine serum	Your choice	
Glutamax supplement (100X)	Thermo Fisher	35050061
Penicillin: Streptomycin solution 100X, Corning	VWR	45000-652
DPBS(+)	VWR	45000-430
Methanol	VWR	BDH1135-4LG
Hoechst 33342	VWR	80056-706
DAPI	VWR	89139-118
Propidium iodide	Thermo Fisher	P3566

Cryopreservation of Mammalian Cells

What should you expect to learn in this lab?

1. Importance of freezing cells
2. The significance of using cryoprotectant in cell freezing

Cryopreservation is the storage of biological materials at extremely low temperatures (–196 °C). At this temperature, all biological activities cease to exist. This allows indefinite storage of biological materials without deterioration over time. Having frozen cell stock minimizes genetic mutations and variations and allows researchers to maintain consistency across experiments.

The success of freezing depends on four critical parameters:

1. Proper handling and gentle harvesting of the cultures
2. Correct use of the cryoprotective agent
3. Controlled rate of freezing
4. Storage under proper cryogenic conditions

Specially designed vials called **cryovials** are used to freeze cells. These vials are designed to withstand explosion during cell thawing when the temperature of the vial and its contents rise quickly from the liquid nitrogen temperature (–196 °C) to the temperature of the lukewarm water (about 25 to 30 °C) used to thaw cells.

It is important to ensure that healthy, actively dividing cells are frozen for successful freezing and subsequent thaw and recovery. This can be achieved by freezing cells at about 70–75% confluency. Avoid freezing cells when their density is too low or too high.

In today's lab, you are provided with 3T3 cells. You will evaluate the effect of "**good**" freezing by freezing the cells in the presence of 10% DMSO (dimethyl sulfoxide) as a cryoprotectant and "**bad**" freezing without the cryoprotectant. Frozen cells will be thawed and plated next week to determine the success of freezing under the two conditions.

Successful freezing should result in greater than 85% cell recovery after thawing.

Preparation

Each student will prepare one cryovial for freezing cells in the presence of cryoprotectant (DMSO). The team will freeze one vial of cells without DMSO. Using a permanent marker, write the following details on the cryovials.

1. Name of cell line or cell type
2. PDL # or passage # (as applicable)
3. One vial marked "**With DMSO**" (one per student)
4. A second vial marked "**No DMSO**" (one per team)
5. Cell count per vial (do this after you determine the cell count after trypsinization)
6. Today's date
7. Your name or initials
8. Write your initials **on the top of the cryovial cap.** (This is not possible with most commercially available cryovials. A flat cap is required to do this (see supply list below).

Procedure: (see diagram on next page)

1. Mark three 15 ml conical tubes as follows:

   Freezing solution A (one per student)—final composition is DMEM/10% FBS/20% DMSO

   Freezing solution B (one per student)—final composition is DMEM/10% FBS/2X final cell concentration for freezing

   Freezing mixture (one per student)—final composition is DMEM/10% FBS/10% DMSO/1X cell concentration
2. Prepare 5 ml "Freezing solution A" by mixing the following
   a. DMEM basal medium - 3.5 ml
   b. DMSO - 1.0 ml
   c. FBS - 0.5 ml
3. Freezing solution B is composed of a complete medium with twice the cell density desired in the freezing vial. That is, if you plan to freeze the cells at 1×10^6 cells per ml, freezing solution B should have a density of 2×10^6 cells per ml. There are two options for "freezing solution B" as listed below. The course instructor will decide which option to use.

   Option 1—The instructor will provide "freezing solution B" at the desired 2X cell concentration. If this option is used, skip to step 4.

   Option 2—Each student will receive one 3T3 culture plate. Students should trypsinize the cells following the sub-culturing protocol and the cell counting protocol. Once you have determined the total cell number, resuspend the cells in DMEM complete medium containing 10% FBS at twice the desired final concentration of cells in the freezing vial. For example, resuspend the cells at 2×10^6 cells per ml if you plan to freeze cells at a final density of 1×10^6 cells per ml. If, for example, your total cell count in the pellet is determined to be 10 million, resuspend the pellet in 5 ml to obtain a cell density of 2×10^6 cells per ml. This is your freezing solution B.

4. For the regular cell freezing **with DMSO**, mix the contents in "freezing solution B" by gently inverting the tube 3–4 times to ensure uniform cell suspension.
5. Using a P-1000 micropipette, quickly transfer 1 ml of the cell suspension to the tube labeled "freezing mixture" tube (see flowchart below).
6. Using a P-1000 micropipette, measure 1 ml of freezing solution A. Introduce freezing solution A to the cells in the "freezing mixture" tube while mixing the solutions **gently and gradually** (do not add the 1 ml freezing solution A all at once). This is called **progressive mixing.** In this method, DMSO is introduced to the cells progressively to minimize shock to the cells. After adding freezing solution A and freezing solution B, mix the solution in the "freezing mixture" tube well to ensure uniform mixing.
7. Transfer 1 ml of the cell-DMSO mixture from the "Freezing mixture" tube to the cryovial marked "With DMSO". Tighten the cap and transfer the cryovial to the "CoolCell" freezing container (make sure that you have marked the necessary details on the vial and the cap as described in the "preparation" section).
8. For "**No DMSO**" freezing (one vial per team), mix the cells in the "Freezing solution B" tube by closing the cap and inverting the tube 3–4 times. Using a P-1000 micropipette, quickly transfer 500 µl ml of the cell suspension to the cryovial marked "**No DMSO**". To this cryovial, add 500 µl regular complete medium (without DMSO) and pipette up and down 3–4 times to mix the solutions. This vial contains the same number of cells as the vial with DMSO but with no cryo-protectant. Transfer the cryovial to the "CoolCell" freezing container.
9. The CoolCell container will remain in the −20 °C freezer until all students complete their freezing procedure. The Collcell container will then be transferred to the −80 °C freezer. The contents in the cryovials will freeze at a rate of 1 °C/min in the CoolCell container in the −80 °C freezer. Next week, you will thaw and plate your frozen cells to determine the success of freezing.

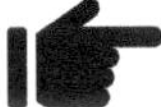

NOTE: Cells frozen at −80 °C will remain viable for many months. However, for long-term storage, vials should be transferred to liquid nitrogen (−196 °C).

Other chemicals used as cryoprotectants are as follows:

1. Glycerol
2. Propylene glycol
3. 2-methyl-2, 4-pentanediol (MPD)
4. Trehalose
5. Sorbitol
6. Diethyl glycol
7. Sucrose
8. Triethylene glycol
9. Polymers (polyvinyl alcohol, PEG, hydroxyethyl starch)

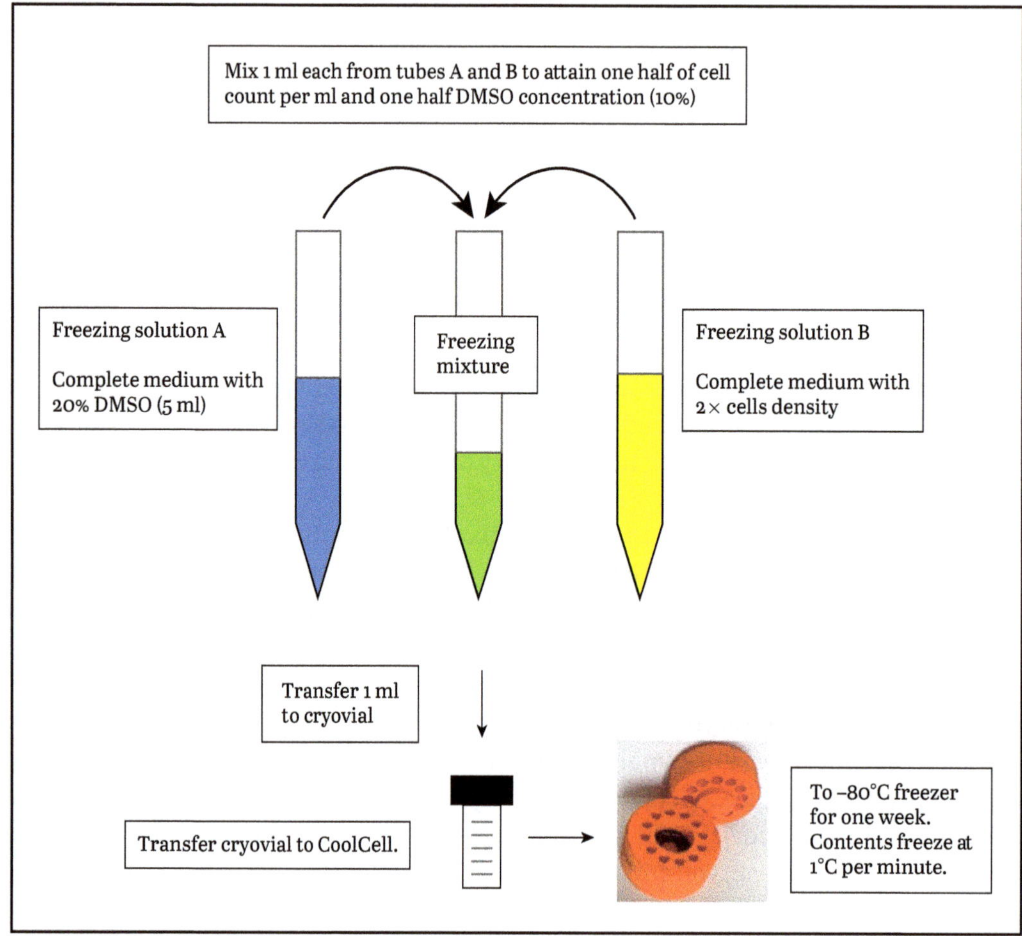

FIGURE BP 4.1 Freezing Mammalian Cells

SUPPLY LIST—This list is for guidance only. Equivalent products may be used based on lab preferences.

Item	Vendor	Catalog #
NIH/3T3 cells	ATCC	CRL-1658
DMEM media (w/4.5 g/L glucose, and sodium pyruvate, no L-glutamine)	VWR	45000-316
Fetal bovine serum	Your choice	
Glutamax supplement (100X)	Thermo Fisher	35050061
Penicillin: Streptomycin solution 100X, Corning	VWR	45000-652
DPBS(−) (without Ca^{++}/Mg^{++})	VWR	45000-434
*CryoELITE cryogenic vial, externally threaded; 2 ml; with writing patch	Fisher Sci	02-912-728
COOLCELL	VWR	95059-860

* The CryoELITE brand of cryogenic vial listed here has a flat cap that allows students to write their initials for easy identification of their vials

Protocol for Thawing and Plating Cells

Thawing of the cells and plating has to be done quickly to lessen the shock to the cells

1. In this process, the frozen cells should be rinsed first to remove the DMSO before seeding into new plates.
2. Take one 15 ml conical tube per cryovial (good freeze and bad freeze) and add 9 ml fresh complete medium to each tube. Keep it aside in the hood.
3. Fill a small beaker with lukewarm tap water. The level of water should not exceed about three quarters of the height of the cryovial.
4. Take the frozen vial of cells from the –80 °C freezer or liquid N2 tank (as applicable) and place it in the beaker containing lukewarm water. Make sure that the vials are standing upright and not floating. This is done to prevent the possibility of tap water from entering the vial. **Complete thawing occurs in about 1–2 min**.

CAUTION: make sure that the contents are completely thawed. During the freezing process, most of the cells would have settled to the bottom and remain trapped in the ice crystals at the bottom of the vial

---

5. As soon as the contents of the vial are completely thawed, take the vial out of lukewarm water container and wipe the outside of the vial dry with a paper towel sprayed with 70% isopropanol. Bring the vial into the hood. Isopropanol can potentially erase the writing on the vial. Therefore, please make sure to properly identify the vial and its contents prior to wiping with isopropanol.
6. Using a P-1000 pipette, transfer the thawed contents of each vial to the corresponding 15 ml tube containing 9 ml fresh complete medium. Rinse the vial a couple of times using 1 ml medium from the same 15 ml tube to which you transferred the cells. This ensures that any remaining frozen cells at the bottom of the vial are recovered. Close the cap of the 15 ml tube and mix the contents in the 15 ml tube by gently inverting it a few times.
7. Spin the tube at 200–250G for 7–10 min.

8. While the tubes are spinning, label 60 mm plates with details for cells from each cryovial. Add 4 ml DMEM complete medium to the plates.
9. After centrifugation, check the size and quality of the cell pellet for the good and the bad freeze. Note the observations in your lab notebook.
10. Aspirate the supernatant leaving less than 0.5 ml of medium with the cell pellet.
11. Using a P-1000 pipette, add 1 ml complete medium to each pellet and resuspend the pellets thoroughly. Transfer the entire content to the labeled 60 mm plate containing 4 ml complete medium. Mix the contents in the plate for uniform distribution of cells.
12. Transfer the plate to the incubator and allow 15–20 min for the cells to settle down.
13. After the 15–20 min of incubation, observe the plates under the microscope and image the cells.
14. Note your observations about the quantity and quality of cells for the "good freeze" and the "bad freeze".
15. Transfer the plates to a 37 °C incubator and let them incubate overnight.
16. On the following day, check both plates under the microscope and specifically check for dead and floating cells. Image the cultures. Fewer floating and dead cells indicate successful freezing and thawing. A good freezing technique is expected to yield greater than 85% cell survival rate. Almost 100% of cells from the bad freeze should be dead and floating.

Alternative Method

If you freeze fewer than 100,000 cells per vial, cell recovery after the initial wash described above may be extremely low. A cell pellet may not be visible after centrifugation. In that situation, you may follow this protocol.

1. Add 4 ml complete media into 60 mm culture plate(s) and label them accordingly.
2. Thaw the cell vial as explained above (steps 3–5).
3. As soon as the contents of the vials are completely thawed, using a P-1000 pipette, transfer the entire contents from the vial (approximately 1 ml) to the 4 ml medium in the 60 mm plate. Rinse the vial using 1 ml medium from the same plate to retrieve any remaining cells in the vial. Add it to the 60 mm plate. Mix the cells in the plate by gently rotating the plates for uniform distribution.
4. Transfer the plate to the incubator and allow 15–20 min for the cells to settle down.
5. After 15–20 min of incubation, observe the plates under the microscope and image the cells.
6. Let the plates incubate for about 3 hours to allow the cells to settle and attach to the plate.
7. After the 3-hr incubation, aspirate the medium from the plates to remove the DMSO still present in the culture medium. Add 5 ml fresh complete medium. Transfer the plate to the 37 °C incubator for overnight incubation and imaging as explained in step 16 above.

3D Cell Culture of Cells

What should you expect to learn in this lab?

1. What is 3D cell culture
2. Properties and characteristics of 3D gels
3. Promises and limitations of 3D gel systems

Materials Provided

1. 1.2 ml of Type I bovine collagen (PureCol EZ, Advanced Biomatrix) in a 1.5 ml tube on ice in the ice bucket. One tube per student.
2. Mouse 3T3 cells constitutively expressing green fluorescent protein (GFP).
   a. A sterile 1.5 ml centrifuge tube containing 100 µl 3T3-GFP cell suspension (250,000 cells total) for one 3D well.
   b. A sterile 1.5 ml centrifuge tube containing 500 µl 3T3-GFPcell suspension at 10,000 cells/ml per one well for regular 2D culture (5,000 cells total).
3. One 15 ml tube containing complete medium for 3T3-GFP cells
4. One 24-well plate per team
5. Pipettes and pipette tips

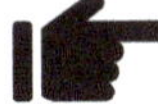

NOTE: PureCol EZ should always be stored on ice. Once you are ready, work quickly to mix the hydrogel and cells in 1.5 ml tubes to avoid gelation of the hydrogel in the tube or the pipet tip.

Procedure

1. Mark the 24-well plate as shown in the diagram below. Note the well coordinates A1–A6, B1–B6, C1–C6 and D1–D6. Team members should mark their respective wells and note the information in their lab notebook.

	1	2	3	4	5	6
A	3D 250K	2D 5K				
B						
C						
D						

2. Place the two 1.5 ml microcentrifuge tubes containing 3T3-GFP cells (250,000 and 5,000 cells) in the microcentrifuge rack.
3. Using a P-1000 pipet, gently take 900 µl of PureCol EZ from the collagen tube (sitting on ice) and add to the tube containing 250,000 cells. The collagen solution is viscous, and care should be taken to avoid creating air bubbles while pipetting.
4. After adding the collagen into the tube, mix the contents gently and deliberately by repeated pipetting (5–8 times) to create a uniform cell suspension.
5. Transfer the cell-hydrogel mixture (~1,000 µl) into the culture well that is marked for 3D gel per the diagram above.
6. Using a P-1000 pipet, transfer the contents from the second tube (500 µl of 3T3-GFP cell suspension, 5,000 cells) to the corresponding well. This will be the 2D control culture.
7. Transfer the plate to the 37 °C incubator and incubate for about 30–45 min to allow PureCol EZ to gel completely. After the incubation period, check the plate to ensure that the collagen–cell mixture has transformed into a semi-opaque gel.
8. After the collagen has gelled completely, bring the plate to the culture hood. Gently add 500 µl of complete medium to the 3D well.
9. With the help of the instructor or the TA, check the 3D gel for uniform distribution of cells under the fluorescence microscope. Return the plate to the incubator. A uniform distribution of cells through the gel thickness indicates good gelation. Cells settled to the bottom of the well indicates poor gelation. Clumping of cells in one area indicates poor mixing.
10. Image the cells today using the fluorescence microscope (day 0). Image again on days 3 and 5 to monitor their progress. If the fluorescent microscope is not available, image using a phase contrast microscope.
11. Pay attention to characteristics such as cell morphology, proliferation rate, or any other feature that you see distinct from the normal 2D culture. Compare cell confluency between the 2D and 3D gels after 1 week of culture.
12. Image the cells again under the fluorescence microscope during next week's lab (day 7). You may use any screen-capture software to make a video of the 3D distribution of cells in the gel, especially on the z-axis.

13. In your lab report, compare and contrast the benefits and challenges of 3D culture versus 2D culture. In particular, discuss cell density, cell quantification, morphological features, growth dynamics, limits of perfusion, etc.

SUPPLY LIST—This list is for guidance only. Equivalent products may be used based on lab preferences.

Item	Vendor	Catalog #
GFP-labeled NIH/3T3 cells	ATCC	CRL-1658 (GFP modification done in-house)
Type I bovine collagen—PureCol EZ	Advanced Biomatrix	5074-35ML
24-well plate tissue culture-treated plate	Any brand	

Wound Healing/Cell Migration Assay

What should you expect to learn in this lab?

1. Cell migration and wound healing
2. Methods of inhibiting cell proliferation
3. Determining the rate of cell migration using imaging software

Purpose: Wound healing/Cell migration assay is used to determine the ability of cells to migrate into an artificially created wound site in vitro and fill or heal the wound partially or completely within a specified period of time. In this experiment, you will determine the average rate of cell migration and the distance traveled by cells to a wound site over a 24–72-hr period.

Procedure

In this lab, you will create a wound by removing a patch of cells by scraping the cells off a specific area within the plate using a pipette tip.

Each team is provided with two 60 mm plates seeded with A172 glioblastoma cancer cell line with a cell confluency greater than 80% on the day of the procedure. This cell line was chosen because of its ability to migrate (invasiveness). Other cell lines that exhibit migration may be used to substitute for A172 cells. One plate is seeded with regular A172 cells in complete media. The other plate contains A172 cells that have been treated with 10 µg/ml mitomycin-C (MMC) for 3.5 hours the day prior to the lab day. MMC is a chemical that blocks cell proliferation, but allows cells to remain viable and metabolically active for up to 3 weeks in culture.

NOTE: In this procedure, you must properly orient the plate to identify regions to be imaged.

1. Hold the culture plate containing A172 cells parallel to the floor. At the bottom of the plate, draw a line at the top and write "TOP" above the line using a marker as shown Figure BP 7.1. This helps to indicate the orientation of the plate. Draw two sets of vertical lines perpendicular to the top line as shown in Figure BP 7.1 (thick dark lines). Each set should be well separated on either side of the midline. Within each set of parallel markings, the lines should be separated by about 5 mm. The lines allow the identification of wound areas for subsequent imaging.

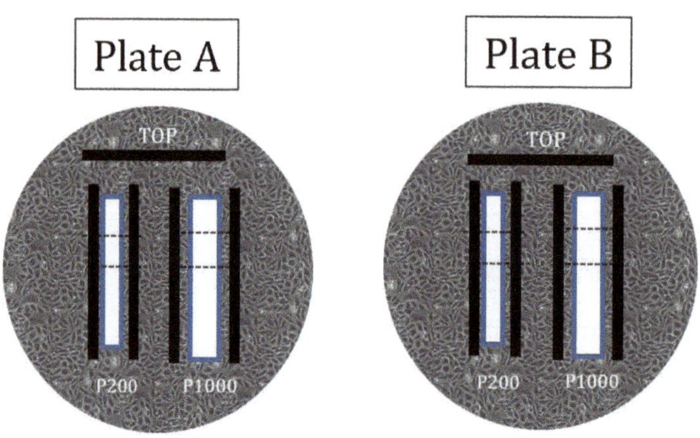

FIGURE BP 7.1 Wound healing

2. **Creating the wound:** Use one sterile P-200 tip and one sterile P-1000 pipette tip to make the "wound". **<u>The following steps should be done quickly to prevent the cells from drying out</u>.**
3. Aspirate culture medium from the plate. Set the plate down on the surface of the hood.
4. To make a wound using a P200 pipet tip, touch the tip of the pipet tip firmly between the first set of vertical lines. Using a firm but smooth continuous single motion, scrape the cells from the area between the two vertical lines from the top to the bottom (see white patch in Figure BP 7.1).
5. Similarly, create a second wound in the same plate using a P1000 pipet tip to scrape off cells from the second set of vertical lines.
6. Repeat steps 4 and 5 for the second plate.
7. Add 1 ml **DPBS** (+) to the plates and rinse with a gentle rotating motion. Aspirate and discard DPBS(+) and repeat the rinse once more. The DPBS (+) rinse helps remove clumps of scraped cells remaining in the plate.
8. After the removal of DPBS, add 5 ml of complete medium to each plate.
9. Check the plates under the microscope using the 4X or 5X objective to locate the wound areas. Ideally, the wound edges should be straight with clean edges.
10. Identify a small area of the scratch to be imaged. This is done by making two horizontal markings perpendicular to the thick parallel lines along as shown Figure BP 7.1 (thin dashed lines). **<u>You will image the migration of cells within these regions only</u>.**

11. Image the wound area at the markings using the 4X or 5X objective. If you can see the whole breadth of the wound with the 10X objective, you may image using the 10X objective as well. These images represent time point zero.
12. Transfer the plates to the incubator for overnight incubation and further imaging.
13. The following day, image the same areas once again. Note the time points to determine the interval between the time the wound was created (time point zero) and subsequent time points until the wound is closed. Some of the narrow wounds may close by the time of the second image. Some may take longer to close. Some may not close at all. Ideally, imaging should be done at 8, 12 or 24 hour intervals or as time permits. You should monitor the migration/wound healing for up to 48 or 72 hours at regular intervals, as necessary. See Figure BP 7.2 for reference.
14. Using an image analysis software of your choice (ImageJ or equivalent), choose at least three points along the wound edge within the area of interest. Calculate the average distance between the wound edges and the center of the wound. Determine the time taken to close the wound completely. The wound may close completely in the untreated control plate by the second imaging time point.
15. Calculate the size of the wound by measuring the distance between the wound edges along three points along the edge of the wounds. Calculate the distance traveled by the cells from either edge to the center of the wound in the control plate and MMC-treated plate. Calculate the average speed of migration per unit time.

Challenge question—Which treatment do you think would close the wound site—untreated or mitomycin-C-treated cells? Explain why. Discuss which data is pertinent to account for migration and wound healing.

Discuss the importance of MMC treatment. What is MMC and what is its role in cancer treatment?

SUPPLY LIST—This list is for guidance only. Equivalent products may be used based on lab preferences.

Item	Vendor	Catalog #
*A172 cells	ATCC	CRL-1620
DPBS(+)	VWR	45000-430
DMEM, with 4.5 g/L glucose, sodium pyruvate, no L-glutamine	VWR	45000-316
Fetal bovine serum	Your choice	
Glutamax supplement (100X)	Thermo Fisher	35050061
Penicillin: Streptomycin solution 100X, Corning	VWR	45000-652
Mitomycin C	Gold Bio	M-900-25

* Other cell types with migratory ability may be substituted for A172.

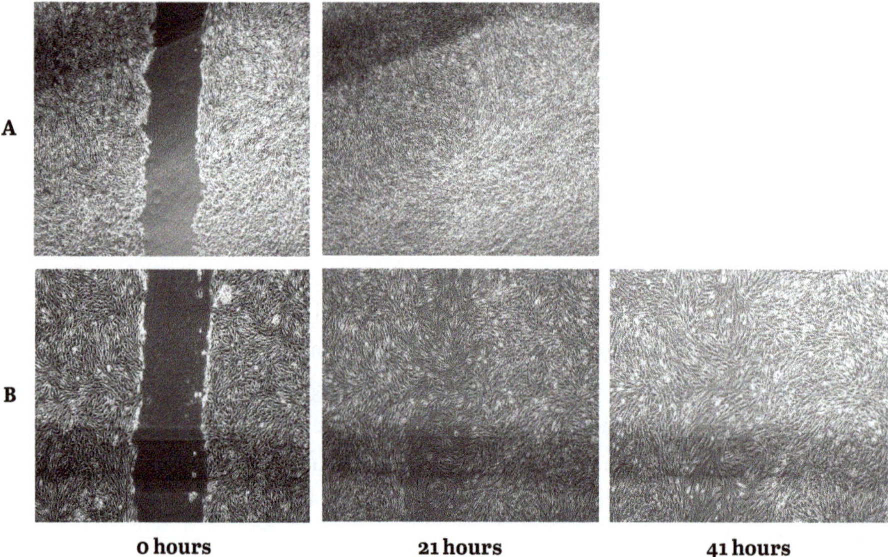

FIGURE BP 7.2 Wound healing/cell migration assay. *Panel A*—untreated control cells without mitomycin-C (MMC) treatment. *Panel B*—cells treated with 10 μg/ml MMC for 3½ hr to prevent cell proliferation. Note that in the untreated control, the wound closes completely by the 21-hr time point (panel A). In the MMC-treated sample, the wound has not completely closed even after 41 hr (panel B). Wound closure in MMC-treated cells can occur only if cells from the wound edge migrate into the wound. As a result, the cell density is much lower around the wound area in MMC-treated plate at the 21 and 41-hr time points. In the untreated plate, wound closure occurs predominantly due to cell proliferation. Therefore, cell density around the wound area in the untreated control remains high

Micropatterning by PDMS Stamping

What should you expect to learn in this lab?

1. What are micropatterns and how they are engineered.
2. Protocols for making micropatterns on glass slides.

Purpose

To introduce students to microcontact printing for basic cell micropatterning techniques.

In this protocol, you will be making only the patterns on the glass slides but **WILL NOT** be culturing cells on the patterns. Therefore, this procedure is performed outside the biosafety cabinet.

Materials Provided

1. Glass microscope slides
2. Pre-made PDMS stamps prepared using photolithography. The micropatterns are either ~200 µm diameter circular patterns or 100 µm square patterns (other patterns may be used based on availability)
3. A mixture of 1% gelatin and 0.05 mg/ml fluorescein prepared in water
4. A pair of forceps
5. 70% isopropanol
6. Slide warmer
7. Pasteur pipette attached to a rubber bulb

Preparation of the PDMS Stamp

1. Take one PDMS stamp and check the side with the micropattern. To do this, place the stamp on a 60 mm plate with the pattern side facing down. Observe under a microscope to confirm the orientation. Take an image.
2. Bring the stamp to the sink. Hold the PDMS piece using a pair of forceps. Clean the PDMS by spraying 70% isopropanol on the pattern side. Rinse the stamp under running cold tap water.

3. Using a paper towel, mop the water on all sides except the pattern side. Keep track of the orientation of the pattern side.
4. Attach a Pasteur pipet to the rubber bulb provided. Hold the stamp using forceps and blow air using the bulb on the pattern surface to air dry the pattern.
5. After air drying, use a piece of scotch tape to stick to the micropattern and peel repeatedly to pick up any fibers or dust from the pattern.
6. Take a new piece of scotch tape and cover the pattern side to prevent dust from settling on the pattern.
7. Place the stamp on a 35 mm or 60 mm plate with the pattern side facing up with the scotch tape covering the surface.
8. Bring the dish to the oxygen plasma cleaner. The instructor or TA will provide instructions to perform plasma treatment of the PDMS stamp. Parameters used to perform plasma oxygen treatment will depend on the type of plasma cleaner in the lab. Remove the scotch tape from the PDMS piece and place the plate with the pattern side facing up. Apply plasma treatment for about 1–2 min to make the pattern hydrophilic. After plasma cleaning, cover the dish and bring the stamp to the bench.

Stamping Procedure

1. You are provided with a 1% gelatin–fluorescein mixture in a petri dish placed on ice
2. Using the forceps pick up the plasma-treated PDMS stamp.
3. Gently touch the pattern side to the gelatin mixture in the petri dish.
4. Place the PDMS piece on a paper towel in a tilted position to drain excess gelatin solution from the surface of the PDMS piece. Take care not to touch the pattern side.
5. Bring the PDMS piece to the slide warmer set at 37 °C. Incubate the PDMS piece with the pattern side facing up for 15 min (or more) until the pattern dries completely. Gelatin, when dried, will form a thin coating on the pattern.
6. After the incubation, pick up the PDMS piece using the forceps. Keep track of the pattern side.
7. **DO NOT RUSH THROUGH THIS STEP.** Take a clean glass slide. Carefully, place the coated PDMS stamp with the pattern side down onto the glass slide. Press down gently and evenly. Avoid air bubbles. DO NOT shift PDMS once it is placed on the glass slide as this could cause streaking and ruin the micropattern.
8. Let the PDMS stay on the slide for about 2 min. This step transfers the gelatin layer representing the micropattern to the glass slide.
9. Before removing the PDMS piece, mark around the stamped area using a marker on the bottom side of the glass slide.
10. Using the forceps, gently peel the PDMS stamp off the stamped surface. Do this by lifting the PDMS piece straight up.
11. **Observe the micropatterns under a fluorescent microscope. Image the patterns using the 5X, 10X, or 20X objective.**
12. Use appropriate imaging software to calculate the size and surface area of the micropattern.

13. If you are not satisfied with your micropattern, repeat the procedure until you obtain good intact micropatterns.

SUPPLY LIST—This list is for guidance only. Equivalent products may be used based on lab preferences.

Item	Vendor	Catalog #
Gelatin from porcine skin	Millipore Sigma	G1890-100G
Fluorescein sodium salt	Millipore Sigma	F6377-100G
Microscope slides	Any brand	

Transfection of Mammalian Cells Using Plasmid DNA

What should you expect to learn in this lab?

1. What is transfection?
2. Understand the importance of plasmid vectors for gene expression analysis
3. Use of lipofection for DNA transfection
4. Utility of fluorescence proteins in gene expression studies
5. Image analysis

Supplies (see vendors and catalog numbers listed in the table at the end of this protocol)

a. Required PPE (lab coat, gloves, safety goggles)
b. One 4-well plate per student, two wells seeded with 50,000 cells, and two wells seeded with 100,000 cells of SK-N-AS cells. In our experience, this cell line provides higher transfection efficiency and higher intensity of green fluorescent protein expression compared to other commonly used cell lines.
c. Viafect lipofection reagent (Promega)
d. pAcGFP plasmid vector stock, 1 µg/µl in Tris-EDTA buffer, pH 8.0.
e. Serum-free basal DMEM medium in 1.5 ml microcentrifuge tube
f. Complete culture media in a 15 ml tube
g. Hoechst nuclear stain (0.5 µg/ml in DPBS(+)) in a 15 ml tube covered with aluminum foil
h. Pipettes, pipette tips, timer, sterile microcentrifuge tubes

1. Check the 4-well plate under the microscope and check for the health of cells. You will be using two wells (one well each of 50,000 and 100,000 cells) for plasmid transfection and the remaining two wells as untransfected controls. Using a marker, mark the wells accordingly and return the plate to the incubator.

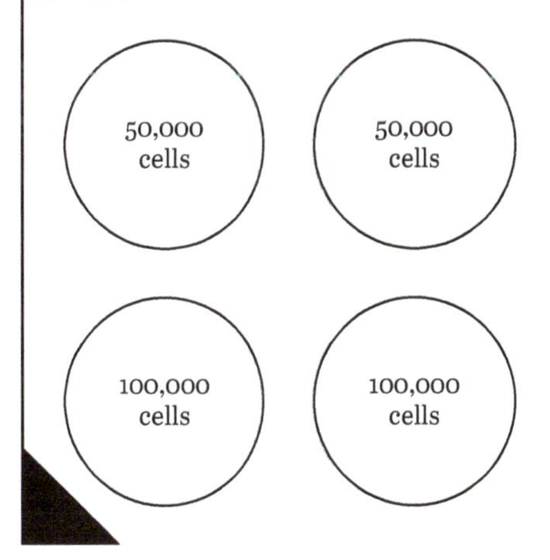

FIGURE BP 9.1 Transfection of Mammalian Cells Using Plasmid DNA

2. Transfer the serum-free media tube from ice to the microfuge tube rack. Allow the contents to equilibrate to room temperature for about 10–15 min.
3. Transfer 100 µl serum-free medium to a sterile 0.5 ml tube. Add 4 µl of pAcGFP plasmid (4 µg total) and mix by pipetting using the P-200 micropipette or by gently flicking the tube. Touch-spin the tube briefly to bring the contents down.
4. Add 8 µl ViaFect reagent to the medium/DNA mixture (ViaFect to DNA ratio of 2:1). Using the P-200 pipette set at 100 µl, **gently** mix the contents by pipetting about 5–6 times. Alternatively, the mixing can be done by **gently** flicking the tube. Touch-spin the tube briefly to bring the contents down.
5. Let the mixture incubate at room temperature in the tube rack inside the hood for 20 min. During this period, the positively charged transfection reagent will form micelles enclosing the plasmid DNA. During transfection, the micelles will fuse with the cell membrane and deliver the DNA to the cells.

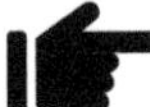

NOTE: Do not pipette the DNA/ViaFect mixture after incubation and right before adding it to the cells. Mixing will disrupt the micelles and result in poor transfection efficiency.

6. After the 20-min incubation, add 50 µl of the transfection mixture to the two wells marked for transfection, each containing 500 µl complete medium.
7. Mix the contents in the wells by gently swirling of the plate.
8. Transfer the plate to the incubator. Allow 24–48 hr for the transfection to proceed and for the cells to express the green fluorescent protein.
9. When it is time to analyze the transfection efficiency and GFP expression, aspirate the medium from the wells and add 500 µl of the 0.5 µg/ml Hoechst stain to the wells. Incubate the plate for 15–20 min in the incubator.
10. Aspirate the contents in the well, add 500 µl of fresh complete medium, and proceed to image the cells.
11. Check the wells under the fluorescence microscope. Visualize and image GFP expression using the filter for green fluorescence and Hoechst nuclear stain using the filter for blue fluorescence. See Figure BP 9.2 for reference. Cells in the untransfected wells will not exhibit fluorescence.
12. Using ImageJ or other similar image analysis programs, calculate the transfection efficiency and the nucleocytoplasmic ratio of the cells.

SUPPLY LIST—This list is for guidance only. Equivalent products may be used based on lab preferences.

Item	Vendor	Catalog #
SK-N-AS cells	ATCC	CRL-2137
4-well plate	VWR	62407-068
DPBS(+)	VWR	45000-430
ViaFect transfection reagent	Promega	E4981
pAcGFP1 Vector	Takara Bio	632468
Hoechst 33342	VWR	80056-706

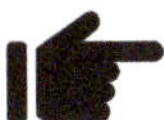

NOTE: Other mammalian cell lines such as HeLa, 3T3, CHO, HEK, Kelly, 293T cells, etc. may be used with varying efficiencies. In our hands, SK-N-AS cells and Kelly cells yielded the best results, especially in a laboratory course setting.

Other lipofection reagents from other vendors may be used. Please adjust the protocol as per the manufacturer's recommendations.

AcGFP protein exhibits cytoplasmic expression. Similarly, nuclear-localized or organelle-localized GFP or RFP may be used depending on the preferences of the course instructor(s).

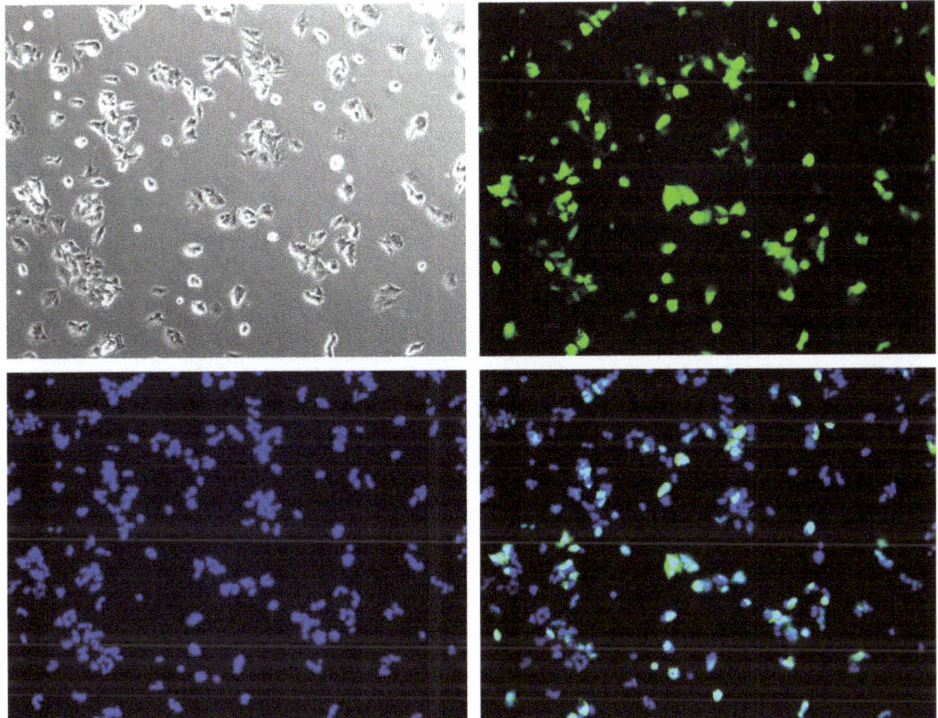

FIGURE BP 9.2 KELLY cells transfected with pAcGFP plasmid DNA expressing green fluorescent protein (GFP) on day 7 after transfection and 5 days after initiation of G418 antibiotic selection to kill off untransfected cells. The majority of the cells express GFP because of the antibiotic selection. Note the variations in the degree of GFP expression in the positive cells. Single clone isolation can be performed to select cells with the desired level of GFP expression. Images in the panel represent phase contrast images of KELLY cells (top left), GFP-expressing transfected cells (top right), Hoechst-stained nuclei (bottom left), and an overlay of GFP and Hoechst images

Differentiation Protocols

C2C12 Differentiation Protocol

What should you expect to learn in this lab?

1. What are C2C12 cells and what are their properties?
2. Factors that contribute to the proliferation and differentiation of C2C12 cells *in vitro*.
3. What are the morphological properties of myofibers produced by fusion of C2C12 cells?

C2C12 is a mouse myoblast cell line that has the potential to differentiate to form contractile myotubes that expresses characteristic muscle proteins. Treatment with bone morphogenic protein 2 (BMP-2) causes a shift in the differentiation pathway from myoblasts to osteoblasts. These cells can remain in a proliferative stage and then be induced to differentiate into contractile myoblasts due to a combination of high confluency and withdrawal from proliferation. To determine the influence of cell density on differentiation efficiency, C2C12 cells were seeded at different densities a day prior to the start of differentiation. It is expected that one of the densities will yield optimal differentiation over a period of 5–7 days after initiation of differentiation.

Supplies

C2C12 proliferation medium—DMEM/10% FBS/1X Glutamax/1% Penicillin–Streptomycin mix
C2C12 differentiation medium is prepared as follows:

Component	Stock concentration	For 10 ml	Final concentration
Adult horse serum	100%	200 µl	2%
ITS	100%	100 µl	1%
Glutamax	100X	100 µl	1X (2 mM)
PennStrep	100X	100 µl	1X (1%)
DMEM basal medium	NA	9.5 ml	
Total volume		**10.0 ml**	

Important Notes

ATCC.org suggests that C2C12 cultures must not be allowed to become confluent as this will deplete the myoblastic population in the culture.

The proliferation medium used here consists of DMEM with high glucose, supplemented with FBS, Glutamax, and penicillin/streptomycin mix. This is the same medium used for culturing NIH/3T3 cells in this course.

The cells are forced to switch from a highly proliferative state to a quiescent state by switching from proliferative to differentiation medium. The differentiation medium contains 2% adult horse serum instead of 10% fetal bovine serum. The addition of insulin via the addition of ITS mix (Insulin/Transferrin/Selenium mix) helps myogenic differentiation.

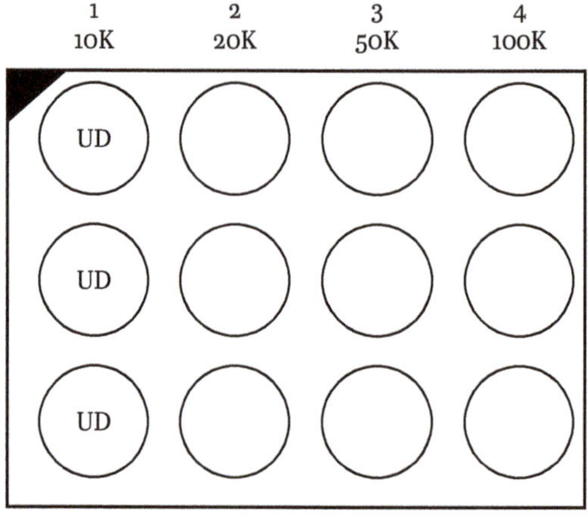

FIGURE DP 1.1 C2C12 Myogenic Differentiation Protocol

Materials Provided

C2C12 cells in 12-well plate per team at the densities shown in Figure DP 1.1.

C2C12 proliferation medium

C2C12 differentiation medium

Procedure

1. Each team will receive one 12-well plate seeded with C2C12 cells. Each student will be in charge of one row of cells per plate.
2. The C2C12 cells are in proliferative media in the 12-well plate (plated yesterday) at the densities shown in Figure DP 1.1 (10,000, 20,000, 50,000, and 100,000) in wells in columns 1, 2, 3 and 4 respectively. Cells in column 1 are "no differentiation" controls. Cells in columns 2, 3, and 4 will be differentiated.
3. Each student will perform steps 4, 5, and 6 for their respective wells.
4. Using vacuum suction, aspirate complete media from wells in columns 2, 3, and 4. Leave column 1 untouched as these are not going to be differentiated.
5. Gently add 1 ml of 1X DPBS (+) to the wells and rinse by gently swirling. Aspirate DPBS+.
6. Add 1 ml of differentiation media per well in columns 2, 3, and 4 to each student's respective wells.
7. Image one row of cells today using the 10X objective (10, 20, 50, and 100K cells). Image the center of the well to obtain sharp images. All students sharing the 12-well plate may share the images since all the wells with different cell densities should look about the same. These images will be your day 0 images.

8. Transfer the plate to the incubator. The cells will differentiate over the next several days and form myofibers.
9. On day 3, image all your wells using the 10X objective. Check to see if fiber-like structures (myofibers) are starting to form in the differentiation wells. The frequency of cell fusion and fiber formation is influenced by initial cell seeding density.
10. The next step is media exchange in all the wells.

CAUTION: Do not use vacuum suction to aspirate media today. The cells would have started differentiation to myofibers. Physical stimulation due to shear force during pipetting can induce contraction of cells causing them to lift off the plate.

Instead of vacuum suction, use a P-1000 pipet to aspirate media and discard the aspirated media into a collection vessel.

Care should be taken to add fresh media VERY GENTLY ALONG THE SIDE OF EACH WELL.

---

11. Perform media exchange in the wells in column 1 by aspirating the old media and adding 1 ml of fresh **proliferatiive media**.
12. Perform media change in wells in columns 2, 3, and 4 by aspirating the old media and adding 1 ml of fresh **differentiation media**.
13. On day 5, image all your wells using the 10X objective. There is no need to make media changes on day 5.

In the Next Lab Session (Day 7 Post-differentiation)

Be very gentle with the cells in this procedure. Mechanical stimulation caused by the pipetting of fluids can induce differentiated and mature myofibers (skeletal muscles) to contract. Powerful contractile forces can lift cells off the plate and be lost.

Day 7: You may opt for two approaches

Option 1:
Fix the cells using cold methanol and image cells under phase contrast using the 10X objective.

1. Aspirate the medium from the wells. Rinse the wells once using 1 ml DPBS(+), aspirate, and discard.
2. Add 1 ml ice-cold methanol to each well. Incubate at room temperature on the bench for 10 minutes.
3. Aspirate and discard methanol and add 1 ml DPBS(+) containing 0.5 µg/ml Hoechst to the wells.
4. Stain for 10 minutes, aspirate the staining solution and add fresh DPBS (+) without Hoechst.
5. Image the wells using phase contrast and blue fluorescence.

Option 2:

Perform live staining of cells using Hoechst nuclear stain and observe the cells under an inverted fluorescence microscope. If there is robust differentiation, you may be able to observe several foci within the wells that exhibit twitching of the myofibers. You may capture the twitching motions either by means of an imaging software or by doing a screen capture of the twitch using an appropriate screen capture software such as Camtasia Studio.

1. You are provided with complete media containing 2 µg/ml Hoechst nuclear stain.
2. Bring the plate into the biosafety cabinet.
3. Using the P-1000 pipette, add 1 ml of media with Hoechst to the 1 ml of media in each well. Now you have 2 ml medium per well with a final concentration of 1 µg/ml Hoechst
4. Allow the staining to proceed for 15–20 min in the incubator.
5. Check for bright blue nuclear fluorescence under a fluorescence microscope.
6. Successful differentiation results in about 50% of the cells aligning and fusing to form multinucleated myofibrils. See Figure DP 1.2 for reference.
7. Watch for patches of contracting myofibers in the culture. You can video capture or screen capture the contractions with appropriate software.

Observations and Analysis

1. Determine which starting density yielded the best differentiation. Discuss the reasons in your lab report.
2. Discuss the significance of the composition of differentiation media in inducing differentiation in C2C12 cells.
3. Did you lose cells during media change? If yes, troubleshoot the problem. Describe how you will overcome this if you have to repeat the experiment.
4. Is there a way to quantify your results? If so, discuss that in your lab report.
5. Did you observe variations in the degrees of differentiation amongst the members within your lab group? Discuss that in your lab report.

SUPPLY LIST

Item	Vendor	Catalog #
C2C12 cells	ATCC	CRL-1772
12-well plate	VWR	62406-165
DMEM media (w/4.5 g/L glucose, and sodium pyruvate, no L-glutamine)	VWR	45000-316
Fetal bovine serum	Your choice	
Glutamax supplement (100X)	Thermo Fisher	35050061
Penicillin: Streptomycin solution 100X, Corning	VWR	45000-652
Donor horse serum	VWR	45001-058
Corning Insulin-Transferrin-Selenium (ITS) 100x Growth Supplement	VWR	45001-090
DPBS(+)	VWR	45000-430
Hoechst 33342	VWR	80056-706

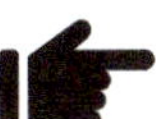

NOTE: The supply list provided here is for guidance only. Equivalent products may be used based on the preferences of each lab.

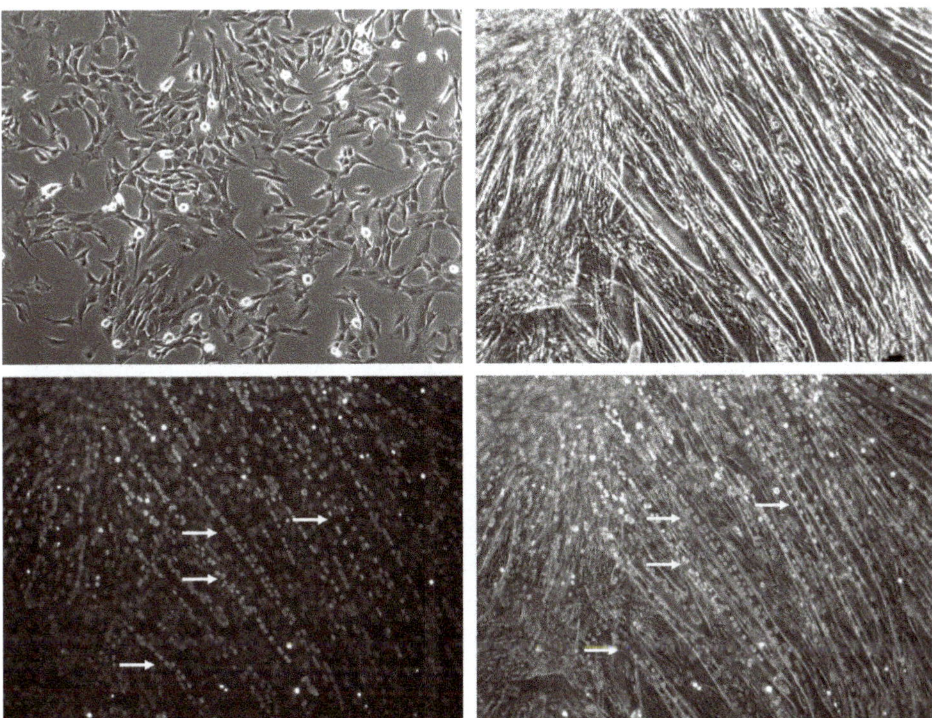

FIGURE DP 1.2 Differentiation of C2C12 cells. Undifferentiated and proliferating cells (top left), formation of long myofibers on day 8 of differentiation (top right), DAPI-stained nuclei of differentiated cells showing multinucleated myofiber (bottom left) and an overlay of myofibers and DAPI-stained nuclei (bottom right). Notice the alignment of nuclei along the length of the myofibers indicating the fusion of multiple individual cells (arrows). Images were captured using a Zeiss Axiovert inverted fluorescence microscope (200X magnification)

Images of the Hoechst stained nuclei were captured using a phase contrast ring to obtain black and white images for better clarity.

Differentiation of Neuroscreen-1 Cells on Various Surface Coatings

---

Objectives

To explore the effect of different substrate coating on the differentiation of Neuroscreen-1 cells

1. Understand the mechanics of surface coating.
2. Determine the effect of coating on neuroscreen-1 differentiation
3. Cell imaging and morphological analysis

Neuroscreen-1 (NS-1) cells are a subclonal line of PC12 cells and are widely used as a standard model system for neurons. NS-1 cells are capable of differentiating to neuron-like cells exhibiting axonal outgrowth in the presence of nerve growth factor (NGF). In this lab, you will differentiate NS-1 cells on three different surface coatings in the presence of NGF and determine and quantify their morphological characteristics.

Supplies

1. 24-well tissue culture-treated plate (one per team)
2. Tube #1—NS-1 cells in complete medium **without** NGF at 10,000 cells/ml stock.
3. Tube #2—NS-1 cells in complete medium **without** NGF at 20,000 cells/ml stock.
4. Tube #3—NS-1 cells in complete medium **with** NGF at 10,000 cells/ml stock
5. Tube #4—NS-1 cells in complete medium **with** NGF at 20,000 cells/ml stock
6. Bovine Type I collagen – 100 µg/ml in sterile water
7. Poly L-lysine (PLL) – 0.01% in sterile water
8. Gelatin – 0.2% in sterile water
9. Sterile water

Procedure

1. Mark the 24-well plate as indicated in Figure DP 2.1.
2. Add 500 µl of each coating solution to the marked wells and close the lid.
3. Allow coating to proceed for 1 hr at room temperature inside the hood.

4. After 1 hr of coating, aspirate the solutions from all wells.
5. Rinse the poly L-lysine wells 3 times each with 500 µl of sterile water. **THERE IS NO NEED TO WASH THE OTHER WELLS.**
6. Move the plate to one side of the hood. Air dry the plate inside the hood for 15–20 min or until the wells are completely dry **with the lid open**. The air circulation inside the hood enhances drying. Take care not to pass anything above the plate while the lid is open.
7. Mix the cell suspension by inverting the tubes right before adding cells to the wells. Add 500 µl of NS-1 cells from the respective tubes to the corresponding wells marked for each treatment. 500 µl of cell suspension yields 5,000 cells and 10,000 cells from the 10,000 cells/ml and 20,000 cells/ml stocks, respectively.
8. Transfer the plate to a 37 °C incubator and allow the cells to settle down for about 20 min.
9. Image any two wells today using 10X and 20X objectives. Cells in all the wells should look the same today. Image cells in the center of the well for good contrast. This is time point zero reference. Return the plate to the incubator.
10. Image cells again on day 4 and day 7 using 10X and 20X objectives. Figure DP 2.2 illustrates an example of NS-1 differentiation.
11. Data analysis—Using ImageJ, Cellprofiler, or other appropriate software, measure the average length of axonal processes, cellular dimensions, and area of the cells. Compare the results from the various treatments and write your conclusions. Use at least 20–25 cells per treatment for analysis.

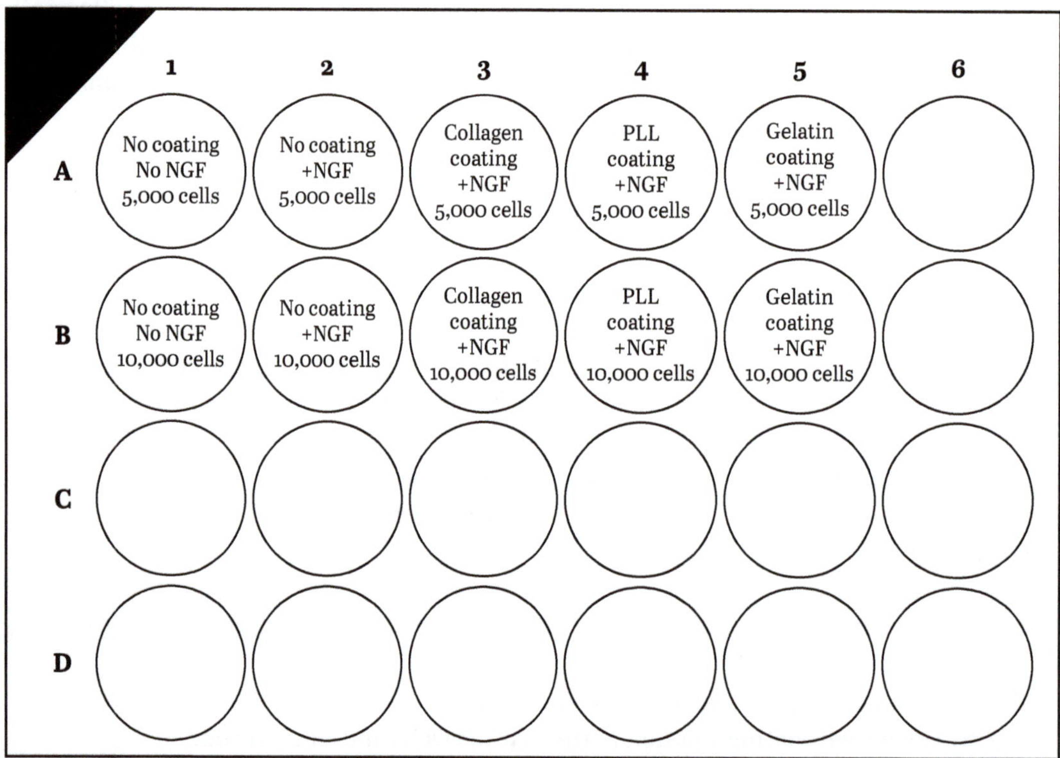

FIGURE DP 2.1 Neuroscreen-1 Cell Differentiation

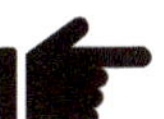

NOTE: Other coating materials may be used at the discretion of the course instructor

SUPPLY LIST: This list is for guidance only. Equivalent products may be used based on lab preferences.
Neuroscreen-1 cell complete medium: RPMI 1640 medium supplemented with 10% horse serum, 10% fetal bovine serum, 1X Glutamax, 1X Sodium pyruvate, and 1X PennStrep, **with and without beta NGF**.

NGF concentrations between 200 to 600 ng/ml can be used. More robust differentiation is observed at higher concentration.

Item	Vendor	Catalog #
Cellomics Neuroiscreen-1 Cells	Thermo Fisher	R04-001
24-Well Plates—Tissue Culture Treated	Any brand	
Sterile Water	Lab supplied	
Bovine Collagen, Type I (PureCol solution)	Advanced Biomatrix	5005-B
Gelatin from Porcine Skin	Millipore Sigma	G1890-100G
Poly-L-Lysine Solution (0.01%)	Millipore Sigma	A-005-C
Beta Nerve Growth Factor, Human Recombinant	Prospec	CYT-579
RPMI 1640, 1X, Without L-Glutamine	VWR	45000-404
Fetal Bovine Serum	Your choice	
Donor Horse Serum	VWR	45001-058
Glutamax supplement (100X)	Thermo Fisher	35050061
Sodium pyruvate	VWR	45000-710
Penicillin: Streptomycin Solution 100X, Corning	VWR	45000-652

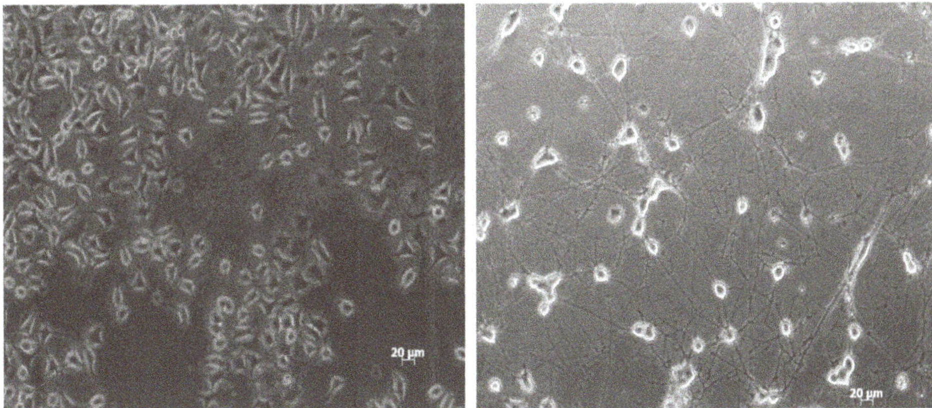

FIGURE DP 2.2 Differentiation of Neuroscreen-1 cells. Phase contrast image of undifferentiated cells (left), and day 7 (right) of differentiation in the presence of 600 ng/ml Nerve Growth Factor. Notice the interconnecting axonal outgrowth in the differentiated cells. Images were captured using a Zeiss Axiovert inverted microscope (200X magnification)

Immunocytochemistry Protocols

Immunocytochemistry Staining for Actin Cytoskeleton Using AlexaFluor-488 Phalloidin

This procedure has been optimized to be completed in about 90 min.
This ICC procedure starting with the cell fixation step can be performed outside the culture hood.

NOTE TO INSTRUCTORS—This protocol was modified to shorten the duration of the procedure to fit into a 2-to-3-hr lab by including quick DPBS(+) rinses between treatments. The typical three rinses for 5 min each are not suitable for large teaching labs. The quick DPBS(+) rinse used in this procedure has worked very well in our laboratory without producing any background fluorescence. Instructors may choose to follow their own standardized procedures in their courses.

What should you expect to learn in this lab?

1. Principles of immunocytochemistry
2. Methods of fixing and permeabilizing cells
3. Fluorescence markers, fluorescence microscopy, and image analysis

Phalloidin is a toxin derived from *Amanita phalloides*, a type of poisonous mushroom (dead cap). Phalloidin has a high affinity for actin cytoskeletal proteins. The use of fluorescently labeled phalloidin allows visualization of the distribution of actin filaments in the cells.

Supplies (see vendors and catalog numbers listed in the table at the end of this protocol)

1. Required PPE (lab coat, gloves, safety goggles). **Students must wear safety goggles** for this procedure because a cell fixative reagent is used. It can cause eye damage in the event of an accidental spill.

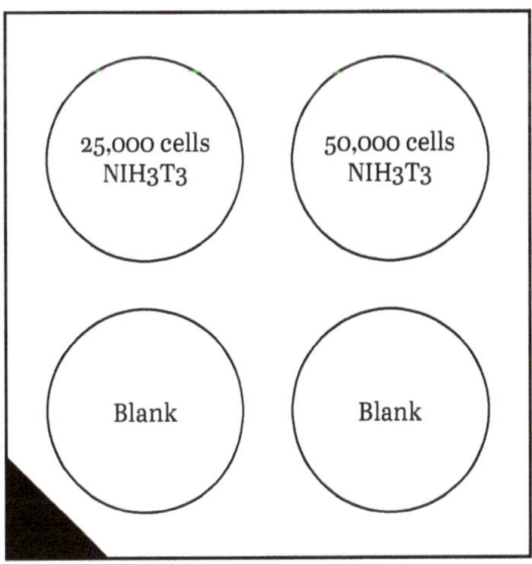

FIGURE I 1.1

2. One 4-well plate per student with 25,000 and 50,000 cells of NIH/3T3 cells seeded the previous day (see Figure I 1.1). Alternatively, all wells may be seeded with cells and two students can share one 4-well plate.
3. 4% methanol-free paraformaldehyde
4. 0.1% Triton X-100
5. 1% Bovine serum albumin (BSA)
6. DPBS with Ca^{++}/Mg^{++} [DPBS (+)]
7. Alexa Fluor 488-conjugated phalloidin diluted in DPBS(+) for green fluorescence or Alexa Fluor 568-conjugated phalloidin diluted in DPBS(+) for red fluorescence.
8. 200 ng/ml DAPI nuclear stain prepared in DPBS(+).
9. Waste collection container and a separate formaldehyde waste collection container

Procedure

1. Check the culture plate under the microscope for the presence and health of the cells and cell confluency. It is best if the cell confluency is approximately 50% for ease of image analysis. Note the notch on the plates to orient the plate. Different brands have different methods to orient the plate.
2. Remove the culture medium from the wells. This can be done by aspirating the medium using pipette tips, a vacuum suction system, or by decanting into a tray. Decanting is easy and saves pipette tips and time. We will use the decanting method in this protocol.
3. Add 500 µl of DPBS(+) to the side of each well very gently, rinse by gentle swirling, and decant into the waste collection tray. Repeat the DPBS(+) rinse one more time and decant.

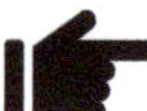

NOTE:

a. It is important to add the solutions very gently to the sides of the wells. Shear forces generated during pipetting can lift the cells off the plate.

b. DPBS(+) must be used in procedures that require multiple rinses because DPBS without Ca^{++}/Mg^{++} can weaken cell attachment and lift the cells off the plate.

---

4. **Fixation step**—Add 500 µl of 4% methanol-free formaldehyde to each well. Incubate at room temperature for 10 min. This procedure fixes the cells but **does not permeabilize the cell membrane.**

The presence of methanol in fixatives can destroy the actin cytoskeleton.

---

5. Using a P-1000 micropipette, aspirate the fixative and **collect it into the formaldehyde waste collection container**. Formaldehyde should not be poured down the drain.
6. Perform two quick rinses using 500 µl of DPBS (+) per well. Using a P-1000 micropipette, **collect these washes into the formaldehyde waste collection tray.**

7. **Permeabilization step**—Add 500 µl of 0.1% Triton X-100 per well. Incubate for 10 min at room temperature. Triton X-100 is a nonionic surfactant that permeabilizes the cells and allows access to antibodies and other reagents to the interior of the cells.

NOTE: High concentrations of Triton X-100 and/or long incubation times can lyse the cells.

8. After Triton X-100 incubation, perform two quick rinses using 500 µl DPBS(+). Decant DPBS(+) into the waste collection tray.
9. **Blocking step**—Add 500 µl of 1% BSA blocking solution to each well. Incubate at room temperature for 10 minutes. BSA is a small sticky protein that will bind to any region on the plate where proteins or molecules such as antibodies (or phalloidin in this case) can bind. BSA coating prevents the nonspecific binding of antibodies and molecules, preventing nonspecific signals.
10. After 10 min of blocking, decant the blocking solution into the waste collection tray.
11. Each student has processed at least two wells so far. You will add the phalloidin reagent to only one well. **It is preferable that the instructor or the TA add the phalloidin to the wells.**
12. **Detection step**—Add 250 µl of Alexa Fluor 488-Phalloidin reagent to one well per student. Incubate for 20 min at room temperature in the dark in one of the drawers to prevent photobleaching. Alternatively, cover the plates with aluminum foil or a suitable cover.

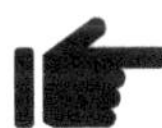

NOTE: Please discuss the importance and relevance of proper experimental controls in research involving immunocytochemistry methods (positive controls, negative controls, etc.)

13. After incubation, decant the phalloidin solution into the waste collection tray. Perform two quick rinses using 500 µl DPBS(+). Decant into the waste collection tray.
14. **Counter staining step**—Add 500 µl of 200 ng/ml DAPI stain prepared in DPBS(+). Incubate for 10 min at room temperature.
15. Decant DAPI stain into the waste collection tray. Add 500 µl DPBS(+) to the well.
16. The plate is ready for microscopy. Image the cells using phase contrast and fluorescence microscopy using filters for Alexa Fluor 488 (green) and DAPI (blue) (see sample image in figure I 1.2). If using Alexa Fluor 568, use the red filter for actin stain.
17. Determine the relevant cellular morphologies, nuclear-cytoplasmic ratios, or other relevant features using appropriate software (e.g., ImageJ).
18. If the plates are to be imaged at a later date, replace DPBS(+) with 500 µl of 0.1% sodium azide. Sodium azide prevents bacterial growth. Seal the plate with parafilm and store it in the fridge.

SUPPLY LIST: This list is for guidance only. Equivalent products may be used based on lab preferences.

Item	Vendor	Catalog #
NIH/3T3 cells	ATCC	CRL-1658
4-well plate	VWR	62407-068
DPBS(+)	VWR	45000-430
Methanol-free paraformaldehyde (10%)	Polysciences	04018
Triton X-100	VWR	EM-TX1568-1
Alexa Fluor 488 phalloidin (green fluorescence)	Thermo Fisher	A12379
Alexa Fluor 568 Phalloidin (red fluorescence)	Thermo Fisher	A12380
BSA, Fraction V (powder)	VWR	RLBSA50
DAPI	VWR	89139-118
Sodium azide	VWR	AA14314-22

Preparation of Alexa Fluor Phalloidin (for the Instructor)

1. Dissolve the contents of the Alexa Fluor phalloidin vial in 1.5 ml methanol.
2. Aliquot in convenient volumes in 0.5 ml microcentrifuge tubes. Store at −20 °C.
3. On the day of the experiment, dilute the methanol stock at a ratio of 1:50 in DPBS(+) or as determined by the instructor. Prepare enough volume based on the number of wells used.
4. Use 200–250 µl of the diluted phalloidin reagent per well in 4-well or 24-well plates.

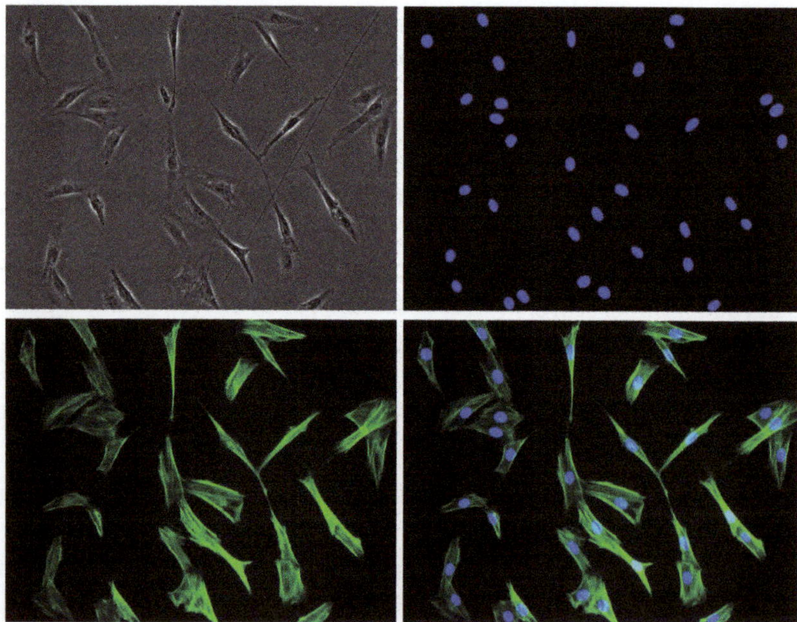

FIGURE I 1.2 Actin cytoskeletal protein staining in 3T3 cells using Alexa Fluor 488-phalloidin. The images represent phase contrast images of 3T3 cells (top left), DAPI-stained nuclei (blue, top right), actin filament stained with Alexa Fluor 488-phalloidin (green, bottom left), and overlay of actin and DAPI stains (bottom right). Images were captured using an inverted Zeiss Axiovert fluorescence microscope (200X magnification)

Immunocytochemistry for Actin Cytoskeleton Using JL20 Actin Antibody

This procedure requires overnight incubation with the primary antibody. It may be shortened to 1 hr and the whole procedure completed on the same day. However, the results may not be optimal. This ICC procedure starting with the cell fixation step can be performed outside the culture hood.

What should you expect to learn in this lab?

1. Principles of immunocytochemistry
2. Methods of fixing and permeabilizing cells
3. Fluorescence markers, fluorescence microscopy, and image analysis

NOTE TO INSTRUCTORS—This protocol was modified to shorten the duration of the procedure to fit into a 2-to-3-hr lab by including quick DPBS(+) rinses between treatments. This procedure has worked very well in our laboratory without any background fluorescence. Instructors may choose to follow their own standardized procedures in their courses.

Supplies (see vendors and catalog numbers listed in the table at the end of this protocol)

1. Required PPE (lab coat, gloves, safety goggles). **Students must wear safety goggles** for this procedure because a cell fixative reagent is used. It can cause eye damage in the event of an accidental spill.
2. One 4-well plate per student with 2 wells seeded with 25,000 and 50,000 cells of NIH/3T3 cells the previous day as shown in Figure I 2.1. Alternatively, all wells may be seeded with cells and two students may share one 4-well plate.
3. DPBS(+)—Dulbecco's phosphate buffered saline with Ca^{++}/Mg^{++}
4. 4% methanol-free paraformaldehyde in DPBS(+)
5. 0.1% Triton-X 100 prepared in DPBS(+)
6. Blocking solution—1% BSA in DPBS(+)

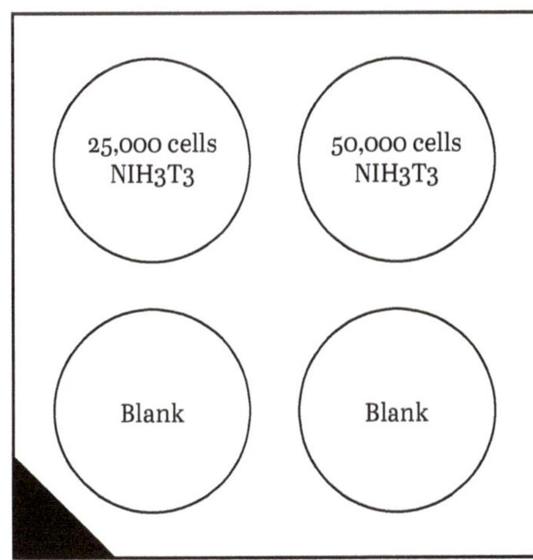

FIGURE I 2.1

7. Antibody dilution buffer—0.05% Tween-20 in DPBS(+)
8. **Primary antibody**—Anti-actin antibody JL20 (mouse) from Developmental Studies Hybridoma Bank or anti-actin antibody from a preferred vendor.
9. **Secondary antibody**—JL20 is a mouse IgM antibody. We will use a goat anti-mouse IgM secondary antibody in this procedure (see supply list). If using a different primary antibody, use the appropriate secondary antibody.
10. 200 ng/ml DAPI nuclear stain prepared in DPBS(+).
11. 0.1% Sodium azide prepared in DPBS(+)

Procedure

1. Check the culture plate under the microscope for the presence and health of the cells and cell confluency. It is best if the cell confluency is approximately 50% for ease of image analysis. Note the notch on the plates to orient the plate. Different brands have different methods to orient the plate.
2. Remove the culture medium from the wells. This can be done by aspirating using pipette tips, a vacuum suction system, or by decanting into a tray. Decanting is easy and saves pipette tips and time. We will use decanting in this protocol.
3. Add 500 µl of DPBS(+) very gently along the side of each well. Rinse by gently swirling. Decant the solution into the waste collection tray. Repeat DPBS(+) rinse one more time and decant.

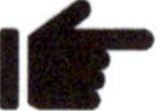

NOTE:

a. It is important to add the solutions very gently to the side of the wells. Shear forces generated during pipetting can lift the cells off the plate.

b. DPBS(+) must be used in procedures that require multiple rinses because DPBS without Ca^{++}/Mg^{++} can weaken cell attachment and lift the cells off the plate.

4. **Fixation step**—Add 500 µl of 4% methanol-free formaldehyde to each well. Incubate at room temperature for 10 min. **This procedure fixes the cells but does not permeabilize the cell membrane.**

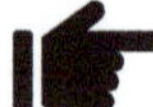

The presence of methanol in fixatives can destroy the actin cytoskeleton.

5. Using a P-1000 micropipette, aspirate the fixative and **collect it into the formaldehyde waste collection container.** Formaldehyde should not be poured down the drain.
6. Perform two quick rinses using 500 µl of DPBS (+) per well. Using a P-1000 micropipette, **collect these washes into the formaldehyde waste collection container.**
7. **Permeabilization step**—Add 500 µl of 0.1% Triton X-100 per well. Incubate for 10 min at room temperature. Triton X-100 is a nonionic surfactant that permeabilizes the cells and allows access to antibodies and other reagents to the interior of the cells.

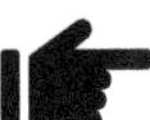

NOTE: High concentrations of Triton X-100 and/or long incubation times can lyse the cells.

8. After Triton X-100 incubation, perform two quick rinses using 500 µl DPBS(+). Decant DPBS(+) into the waste collection tray.
9. **Blocking step**—Add 500 µl of 1% BSA blocking solution to each well. Incubate at room temperature for 10 minutes. BSA is a small sticky protein that will bind to any region on the plate where other proteins such as antibodies can bind. BSA coating prevents the nonspecific binding of antibodies and molecules, preventing nonspecific signals.
10. During the BSA incubation period, prepare the primary antibody reagent by diluting JLA20 primary antibody 1:50 in antibody dilution buffer. If using antibodies from different vendors, follow the manufacturer's instructions for preparing the dilutions and incubation times.
11. After 10 min of blocking, decant the blocking solution into the waste collection tray.
12. **Detection step**—Each student has processed at least two wells so far. You need only one for the detection step. Add 250 µl of the prepared primary antibody per well. Seal the plate using parafilm and incubate overnight at 4 °C in the fridge.

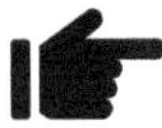

NOTE: Discuss the importance and relevance of proper experimental controls in research involving immunocytochemistry methods (antibody controls, positive controls, negative controls, etc.)

13. The following day, prepare a 1:500 dilution of the secondary antibody in antibody dilution buffer. You may use green or red fluorescing secondary antibody (see supply list).
14. Decant the primary antibody solution into the waste collection tray.
15. Perform three quick rinses using 500 µl of DPBS(+) per well. Decant DPBS(+) into the waste collection tray.
16. Add 250 µl secondary antibody per well. Incubate the plate at room temperature for 60 min in the dark inside a drawer to prevent photobleaching. Alternatively, cover the plates with aluminum foil.
17. After incubation, decant secondary antibody solution and perform three quick rinses with 500 µl of DPBS(+). Decant DPBS(+) into the waste collection tray.
18. **Counter staining step**—Perform counterstaining by adding 500 µl of DAPI nuclear stain per well. Incubate at room temperature for 10 min.
19. Decant the staining solution into the waste collection tray. Add 500 µl fresh DPBS(+) per well. Cells are ready for observation by fluorescence microscopy. Image the cells using phase contrast and fluorescence microscopy using filters for Alexa Fluor 488 (green) and DAPI (blue) (see sample image in Figure I 2.2). If using Alexa Fluor 568, use the red filter for actin stain.
20. If the plates are to be imaged at a later date, replace DPBS(+) with 500 µl of 0.1% sodium azide. Sodium azide prevents bacterial growth. Seal the plate with parafilm and store it in the fridge.

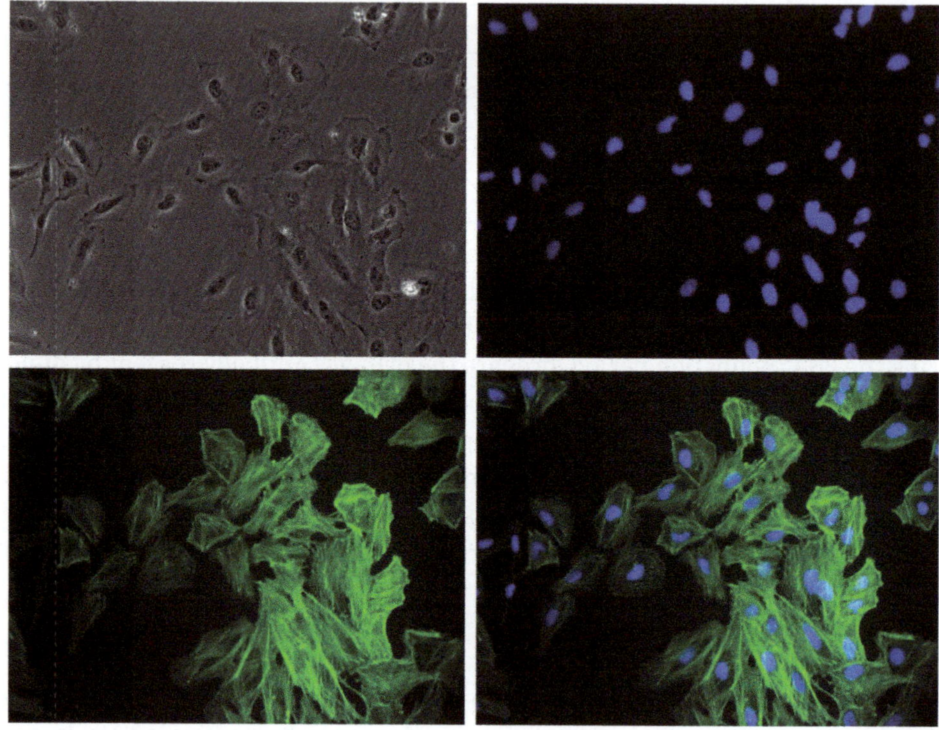

FIGURE I 2.2 Actin cytoskeletal protein staining in HeLa cells using JL20 primary antibody (DSHB). The images represent phase contrast images of HeLa cells (top left), DAPI-stained nuclei (blue fluorescence, top right), actin filament stained with JL20 antibody (green fluorescence, bottom left), and overlay of actin and DAPI stains (bottom right). Images were captured using an inverted Zeiss Axiovert fluorescence microscope (200X magnification)

SUPPLY LIST: This list is for guidance only. Equivalent products may be used based on lab preferences.

Item	Vendor	Catalog #
NIH/3T3 cells	ATCC	CRL-1658
4-well plate	VWR	62407-068
DPBS(+)	VWR	45000-430
Methanol-free paraformaldehyde (10%)	Polysciences	04018
Triton X-100	VWR	EM-TX1568-1
Tween 20	VWR	95059-248
BSA, Fraction V (powder)	VWR	RLBSA50
*Anti-actin primary antibody (Mouse IgM, kappa light chain)	DSHB	JLA-20
*Alexa Fluor® 488 Goat anti-Mouse IgM (Heavy chain) Cross-Adsorbed Secondary Antibody	Thermo Fisher	A-21042
*Alexa Fluor® 568 Goat anti-Mouse IgM (Heavy chain) Cross-Adsorbed Secondary Antibody	Thermo Fisher	A-21043
DAPI	VWR	89139-118
Sodium azide	VWR	AA14314-22

* If you are using an actin primary antibody from a different vendor, use the appropriate secondary antibody.

Immunocytochemistry for Beta Tubulin Cytoskeleton

This procedure requires overnight incubation with the primary antibody. It may be shortened to 1 hr and the whole procedure completed on the same day. However, the results may not be optimal. This ICC procedure starting with the fixing step can be performed outside the culture hood.

What should you expect to learn in this lab?

1. Principles of immunocytochemistry
2. Methods of fixing and permeabilizing cells
3. Fluorescence markers
4. Fluorescence microscopy and image analysis

NOTE TO INSTRUCTORS— This protocol was modified to shorten the duration of the procedure in a teaching lab setting by including quick DPBS(+) rinses between treatments. This procedure has worked very well in our laboratory without any background fluorescence. Instructors may choose to follow their own standardized procedures in their courses.

Supplies (see vendors and catalog numbers listed in the table at the end of this protocol)

1. Required PPE (lab coat, gloves, safety goggles). **Students must wear safety goggles** for this procedure because a cell fixative reagent is used. It can cause eye damage in the event of an accidental spill.
2. One 4-well plate per student with 2 wells seeded with 25,000 and 50,000 cells of NIH/3T3 cells the previous day as shown in Figure I 3.1. Alternatively, all wells may be seeded with cells and two students may share one 4-well plate.
3. DPBS(+)—Dulbecco's phosphate buffered saline (Ca^{++}/Mg^{++})
4. 4% methanol-free paraformaldehyde in DPBS(+)
5. 0.1% Triton-X 100 prepared in DPBS(+)

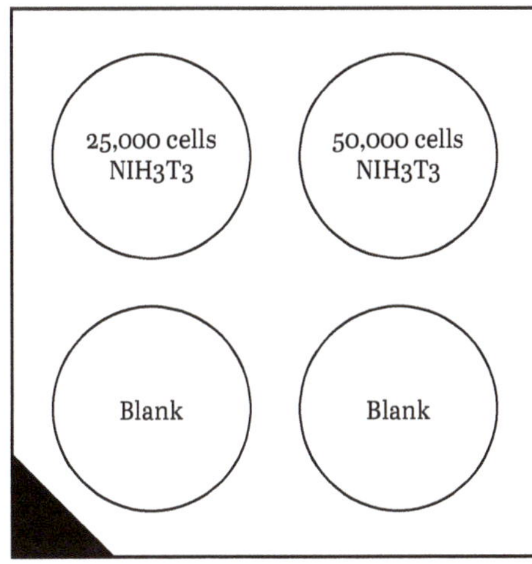

FIGURE I 3.1

6. Blocking solution—1% BSA in DPBS(+)
7. Antibody dilution buffer—0.05% Tween-20 in DPBS(+)
8. **Primary antibody**—Anti-beta tubulin antibody E7 (mouse) from Developmental Studies Hybridoma Bank or anti-beta tubulin antibodies from preferred vendors.
9. **Secondary antibody**—E7 is a mouse IgG1 antibody. We will use a goat anti-mouse IgG1 secondary antibody in this procedure (see supply list). If using a different primary antibody, use the appropriate secondary antibody.
10. 200 ng/ml DAPI nuclear stain prepared in DPBS(+).
11. 0.1% Sodium azide prepared in DPBS(+)

Procedure

1. Check the culture plate under the microscope for the presence and health of the cells and cell confluency. It is best if the cell confluency is approximately 50% for ease of image analysis. Note the notch on the plates to orient the plate. Different brands have different methods to orient the plate.
2. Remove the culture medium from the wells. This can be done by aspirating using pipette tips, a vacuum suction system, or by decanting into a tray. Decanting is easy and saves pipette tips and time. We will use decanting in this protocol.
3. Add 500 µl of DPBS(+) very gently along the side of each well. Rinse by gently swirling. Decant the solution into the waste collection tray. Repeat DPBS(+) rinse one more time and decant.

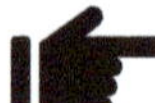

NOTE:

a. It is important to add the solutions very gently to the side of the wells. Shear forces generated during pipetting can lift the cells off the plate.

b. DPBS(+) must be used in procedures that require multiple rinses because DPBS without Ca^{++}/Mg^{++} can weaken cell attachment and lift the cells off the plate.

4. **Fixation step**—Add 500 µl of 4% methanol-free formaldehyde to each well. Incubate at room temperature for 10 min. **This procedure fixes the cells but does not permeabilize the cell membrane.**
5. Using a P-1000 micropipette, aspirate the fixative and **collect it into the formaldehyde waste collection container.** Formaldehyde should not be poured down the drain.
6. Perform two quick rinses using 500 µl of DPBS (+) per well. Using a P-1000 micropipette, **collect these washes into the formaldehyde waste collection container.**
7. **Permeabilization step**—Add 500 µl of 0.1% Triton X-100 per well. Incubate for 10 min at room temperature. Triton X-100 is a nonionic surfactant that permeabilizes the cells and allows access to antibodies and other reagents to the interior of the cells.

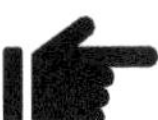

NOTE: High concentrations of Triton X-100 and/or long incubation times can lyse the cells.

8. After Triton X-100 incubation, perform two quick rinses using 500 μl DPBS(+). Decant DPBS(+) into the waste collection tray.
9. **Blocking step**—Add 500 μl of 1% BSA blocking solution to each well. Incubate at room temperature for 10 min. BSA is a small sticky protein that will bind to any region on the plate where other proteins such as antibodies can bind. BSA coating prevents the nonspecific binding of antibodies and molecules, preventing nonspecific signals.
10. During the BSA incubation period, prepare the primary antibody by diluting E7 primary antibody 1:50 in antibody dilution buffer.
11. After incubation with the blocking reagent, decant the blocking solution into the tray.
12. **Detection step**—Each student has processed at least two wells so far. You need only one for the detection step. Add 250 μl of the prepared primary antibody per well. Seal the plate using parafilm and incubate overnight at 4 °C in the fridge.

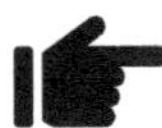

NOTE: Discuss the importance and relevance of proper experimental controls in research involving immunocytochemistry methods (antibody controls, positive controls, negative controls, etc.)

13. The following day, prepare a 1:500 dilution of the secondary antibody in antibody dilution buffer. You may use green or red fluorescing secondary antibody (see supply list).
14. Decant the primary antibody solution into the waste collection tray.
15. Perform three quick rinses using 500 μl of DPBS(+) per well. Decant DPBS(+) into the waste collection tray.
16. Add 250 μl secondary antibody per well. Incubate the plate at room temperature for 60 min in the dark inside a drawer to prevent photobleaching. Alternatively, cover the plates with aluminum foil.
17. After incubation, decant the secondary antibody solution and perform three quick rinses with 500 μl of DPBS(+). Decant DPBS(+) into the waste collection tray.
18. **Counter staining step**—Perform counterstaining by adding 500 μl of DAPI nuclear stain per well. Incubate at room temperature for 10 min.
19. Decant the staining solution into the waste collection tray. Add 500 μl fresh DPBS(+) per well. Cells are ready for observation by fluorescence microscopy. Image the cells using phase contrast and fluorescence microscopy using filters for Alexa Fluor 488 (green) and DAPI (blue) (see sample image in Figure I 3.2). If using Alexa Fluor 568, use the red filter for actin stain.
20. If the plates are to be imaged at a later date, replace DPBS(+) with 500 μl of 0.1% sodium azide. Sodium azide prevents bacterial growth. Seal the plate with parafilm and store it in the fridge.

SUPPLY LIST: This list is for guidance only. Equivalent products may be used based on lab preferences.

Item	Vendor	Catalog #
NIH/3T3 cells	ATCC	CRL-1658
4-well plate	VWR	62407-068
DPBS(+)	VWR	45000-430
Methanol-free paraformaldehyde (10%)	Polysciences	04018
Triton X-100	VWR	EM-TX1568-1
Tween 20	VWR	95059-248
BSA, Fraction V (powder)	VWR	RLBSA50
*Anti-beta tubulin primary antibody (mouse IgG1)	DSHB	E7
*Alexa Fluor® 488 Goat anti-Mouse IgG1 Cross-Adsorbed Secondary Antibody (for green fluorescence)	Thermo Fisher	A-21121
*Alexa Fluor® 568 Goat anti-Mouse IgG1 Cross-Adsorbed Secondary Antibody (for red fluorescence)	Thermo Fisher	A-21124
DAPI	VWR	89139-118
Sodium azide	VWR	AA14314-22

* If you are using beta tubulin antibody from a different vendor, use the appropriate secondary antibody

NOTE: Methanol may be used to fix and permeabilize the cells in one step. If methanol is used for the fixation step (step 4), skip the permeabilization step and continue to step 8 in the above procedure.

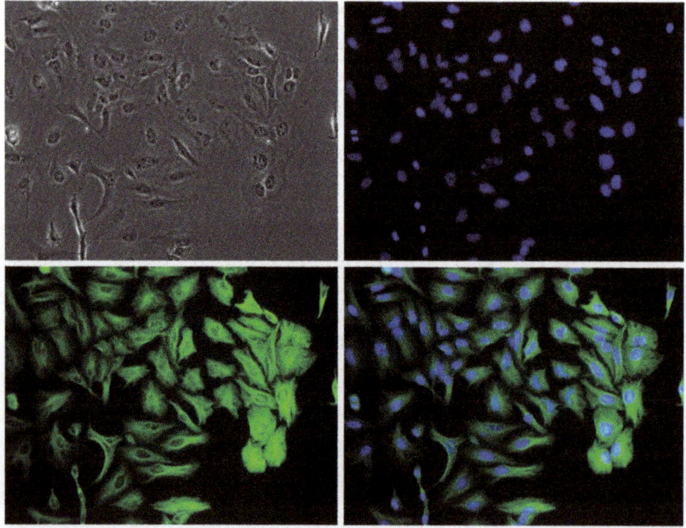

FIGURE I 3.2 Beta tubulin cytoskeletal protein staining in HeLa cells using E7 primary antibody (DSHB). The images represent phase contrast images of HeLa cells (top left), DAPI-stained nuclei (blue fluorescence, top right), beta tubulin filament stained with E7 antibody (green fluorescence, bottom left) and overlay of beta tubulin and DAPI stains (bottom right). Images were captured using an inverted Zeiss Axiovert fluorescence microscope (200X magnification)

Immunocytochemistry to Detect Vimentin

This procedure requires overnight incubation with the primary antibody. The primary antibody incubation time may be shortened to 1 hr and the whole procedure completed on the same day. However, the results may not be optimal. This ICC procedure starting with the cell fixation step can be performed outside the culture hood.

What should you expect to learn in this lab?

1. Principles of immunocytochemistry
2. Methods of fixing and permeabilizing cells
3. Fluorescence markers, fluorescence microscopy and image analysis

NOTE TO INSTRUCTORS—This protocol was modified to shorten the duration of the procedure to fit into a 2-to-3-hr lab period by including quick DPBS(+) rinses between treatments. This procedure has worked very well in our laboratory without any background fluorescence. Instructors may choose to follow their own standardized procedures in their courses.

Supplies (see vendors and catalog numbers listed in the table at the end of this protocol)

1. Required PPE (lab coat, gloves, safety goggles). **Students must wear safety goggles** for this procedure because a cell fixative reagent is used. It can cause eye damage in the event of an accidental spill.
2. One 4-well plate per student with 2 wells seeded with 25,000 and 50,000 cells of NIH/3T3 cells the previous day as shown in Figure I 4.1. Alternatively, all wells may be seeded with cells and two students may share one 4-well plate.
3. DPBS(+)—Dulbecco's phosphate buffered saline (Ca^{++}/Mg^{++})
4. 4% methanol-free paraformaldehyde in DPBS(+)

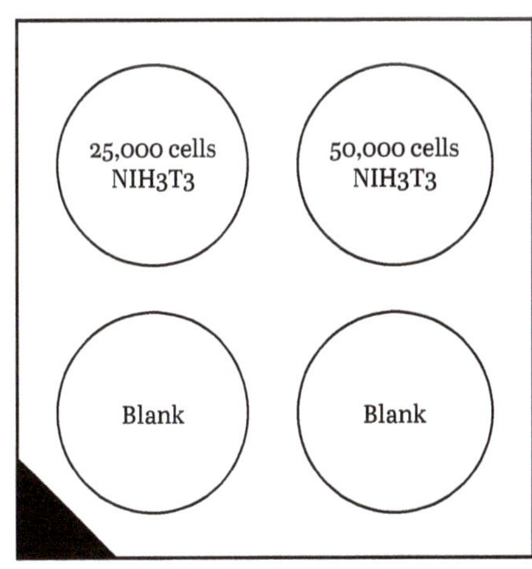

FIGURE I 4.1

5. 0.1% Triton-X 100 prepared in DPBS(+)
6. Blocking solution—1% BSA in DPBS(+)
7. Antibody dilution buffer—0.05% Tween-20 in DPBS(+)
8. **Primary antibody**—Anti-vimentin antibody 40E-C (mouse) from Developmental Studies Hybridoma Bank or anti-vimentin antibodies from preferred vendors.
9. **Secondary antibody**—40E-C is a mouse IgM antibody. We will use a goat anti-mouse IgM secondary antibody in this procedure (see supply list). If using other primary antibodies, use the appropriate secondary antibody.
10. 200 ng/ml DAPI nuclear stain prepared in DPBS(+).
11. 0.1% Sodium azide prepared in DPBS(+)

Procedure

1. Check the culture plate under the microscope for the presence and health of the cells and cell confluency. It is best if the cell confluency is approximately 50% for ease of image analysis. Note the notch on the plates to orient the plate. Different brands have different methods to orient the plate.
2. Remove the culture medium from the wells. This can be done by aspirating using pipette tips, a vacuum suction system, or by decanting into a tray. Decanting is easy and saves pipette tips and time. We will use decanting in this protocol.
3. Add 500 µl of DPBS(+) very gently along the side of the each well. Rinse by gently swirling. Decant the solution into the waste collection tray. Repeat DPBS(+) rinse one more time and decant.

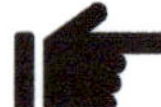

NOTE:

a. It is important to add the solutions very gently to the side of the wells. Shear forces generated during pipetting can lift the cells off the plate.

b. DPBS(+) must be used in procedures that require multiple rinses because DPBS without Ca^{++}/Mg^{++} can weaken cell attachment and lift the cells off the plate.

---

4. **Fixation step**—Add 500 µl of 4% methanol-free formaldehyde to each well. Incubate at room temperature for 10 min. **This procedure fixes the cells but does not permeabilize the cell membrane.**
5. Using a P-1000 micropipette, aspirate the fixative and **collect into the formaldehyde waste collection container.** Formaldehyde should not be poured down the drain.
6. Perform two quick rinses using 500 µl of DPBS (+) per well. Using a P-1000 micropipette, **collect these washes into the formaldehyde waste collection container.**
7. **Permeabilization step**—Add 500 µl of 0.1% Triton X-100 per well. Incubate for 10 min at room temperature. Triton X-100 is a nonionic surfactant that permeabilizes the cells and allows access to antibodies and other reagents to the interior of the cells. Decant after the 10 min incubation.

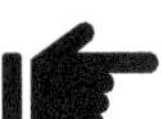

NOTE: High concentrations of Triton X-100 and/or long incubation times can lyse the cells.

8. Perform two quick rinses using 500 µl DPBS(+). Decant DPBS(+) into the waste collection tray.
9. **Blocking step**—Add 500 µl of 1% BSA blocking solution to each well. Incubate at room temperature for 10 min. BSA is a small sticky protein that will bind to any region on the plate where other proteins such as antibodies can bind. BSA coating prevents nonspecific binding of antibodies and molecules, preventing nonspecific signals.
10. During the BSA incubation period, prepare the primary antibody reagent by diluting 40E-C primary antibody 1:50 in antibody dilution buffer. If using antibodies from different vendors, follow the manufacturer's instructions for preparing the dilutions and incubation times.
11. After 10 min of blocking, decant the blocking solution into the waste collection tray.
12. **Detection step**—Each student has processed at least two wells so far. You need only one for the detection step. Add 250 µl of the prepared primary antibody per well. Seal the plate using parafilm and incubate overnight at 4 °C in the fridge.

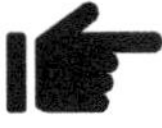

NOTE: Discuss the importance and relevance of proper experimental controls in research involving immunocytochemistry methods (antibody controls, positive controls, negative controls, etc.)

13. The following day, prepare a 1:500 dilution of the secondary antibody in antibody dilution buffer. You may use green or red fluorescing secondary antibody (see supply list).
14. Decant the primary antibody solution into the waste collection tray.
15. Perform three quick rinses using 500 µl of DPBS(+) per well. Decant DPBS(+) into the waste collection tray.
16. Add 250 µl secondary antibody per well. Incubate the plate at room temperature for 60 min in the dark inside a drawer to prevent photo-bleaching. Alternatively, cover the plates with aluminum foil.
17. After incubation, decant secondary antibody solution and perform three quick rinses with 500 µl of DPBS(+). Decant DPBS(+) into the waste collection tray.
18. **Counter staining step**—Perform counterstaining by adding 500 µl of DAPI nuclear stain per well. Incubate at room temperature for 10 min.
19. Decant the staining solution into the waste collection tray. Add 500 µl fresh DPBS(+) per well. Cells are ready for observation by fluorescence microscopy. Image the cells using phase contrast and fluorescence microscopy using filters for Alexa Fluor 488 (green) and DAPI (blue) (see sample image in Figure I 4.2). If using Alexa Fluor 568, use the red filter for actin stain.
20. If the plates are to be imaged at a later date, replace DPBS(+) with 500 µl of 0.1% sodium azide. Sodium azide prevents bacterial growth. Seal the plate with parafilm and store it in the fridge.

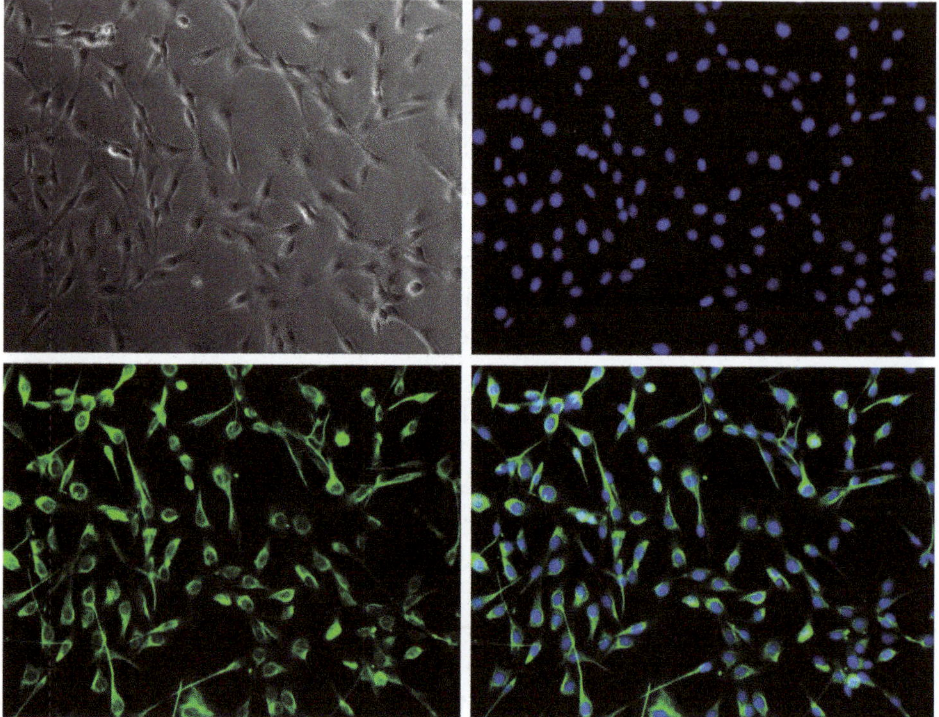

FIGURE I 4.2 Vimentin cytoskeletal protein staining in 3T3 cells using 40E-C primary antibody (DSHB). The images represent phase contrast image of 3T3 cells (top left), DAPI-stained nuclei (blue, top right), vimentin filament stained with 40E-C antibody (green, bottom left), and overlay of vimentin and DAPI stains (bottom right). Notice that vimentin is densely packed around the nucleus of the cells. Images were captured using an inverted Zeiss Axiovert fluorescence microscope (200X magnification)

SUPPLY LIST: This list is for guidance only. Equivalent products may be used based on lab preferences.

Item	Vendor	Catalog #
NIH/3T3 cells	ATCC	CRL-1658
4-well plate	VWR	62407-068
DPBS(+)	VWR	45000-430
Methanol-free paraformaldehyde (10%)	Polysciences	04018
Triton X-100	VWR	EM-TX1568-1
Tween 20	VWR	95059-248
BSA, Fraction V (powder)	VWR	RLBSA50
*Anti-vimentin primary antibody (mouse)	DSHB	40E-C
*Alexa Fluor® 488 Goat anti-Mouse IgM (Heavy chain) Cross-Adsorbed Secondary Antibody	Thermo Fisher	A-21042

*Alexa Fluor® 568 Goat anti-Mouse IgM (Heavy chain) Cross-Adsorbed Secondary Antibody	Thermo Fisher	A-21043
DAPI	VWR	89139-118
Sodium azide	VWR	AA14314-22

* If you are using vimentin primary antibody from a different vendor, use the appropriate secondary antibody.

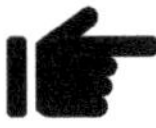

NOTE: Methanol may be used to fix and permeabilize the cells in one step. If methanol is used for the fixation step (step 4), skip the permeabilization step and continue to step 8 in the above procedure.

Immunocytochemistry to Detect Myosin Heavy Chain in C2C12 Cells

This procedure has been optimized for completion in less than 3 hours.
This protocol should be done on differentiated C2C12 cells or a muscle cell type that expresses myosin heavy chain protein. Please refer to the C2C12 differentiation protocol to prepare the cells for this procedure. **Adjust the cell numbers for 24-well plates.**

This ICC procedure **does not require** the use of a culture hood.

This ICC procedure starting with the cell fixation step can be performed outside the culture hood. What should you expect to learn in this lab?

1. Cellular differentiation
2. Principles of immunocytochemistry
3. Methods of fixing and permeabilizing cells
4. Fluorescence markers, fluorescence microscopy, and image analysis

NOTE TO INSTRUCTORS—This protocol was modified to shorten the duration of the procedure to fit into a 2-to-3-hr lab period by including quick DPBS(+) rinses between treatments. This procedure has worked very well in our laboratory without any background fluorescence. Instructors may choose to follow their own standardized procedures in their courses.

Supplies (see vendors and catalog numbers listed in the table at the end of this protocol)

1. Required PPE (lab coat, gloves, safety goggles). **Students must wear safety goggles** for this procedure because a cell fixative reagent is used. It can cause eye damage in the event of an accidental spill.
2. One 4-well plate per student; 2 wells with C2C12 cells differentiated for 5–6 days to express myosin heavy chain and one well with undifferentiated control.
3. DPBS(+)—Dulbecco's phosphate buffered saline with Ca^{++}/Mg^{++}

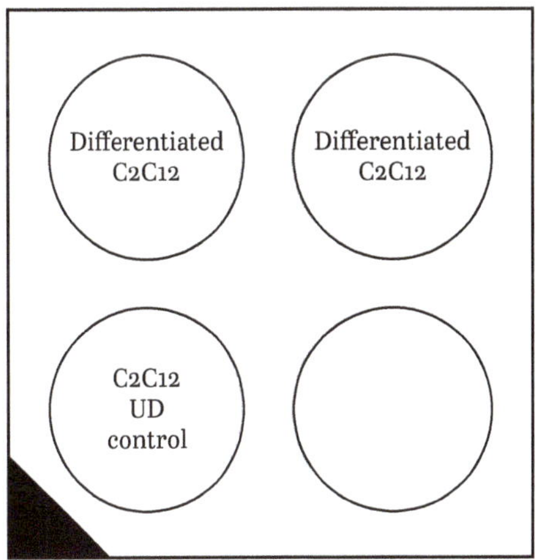

FIGURE I 5.1

4. Ice-cold methanol fixative
5. 0.1% Triton-X 100 prepared in DPBS(+)
6. Blocking solution—1% BSA in DPBS(+)
7. Antibody dilution buffer—0.05% Tween-20 in DPBS(+)
8. **Primary antibody**—Anti-myosin (heavy chain) antibody MF20 (mouse) from Developmental Studies Hybridoma Bank or anti-myosin (heavy chain) antibodies from preferred vendors. Alternatively, other skeletal muscle-specific primary antibodies may be used.
9. **Secondary antibody**—MF20 is a mouse IgG2b antibody. We will use a goat anti-mouse IgG secondary antibody in this procedure (see supply list). If using a different primary antibody, use the appropriate secondary antibody.
10. 200 ng/ml DAPI nuclear stain prepared in DPBS(+).
11. 0.1% Sodium azide prepared in DPBS(+)

Procedure

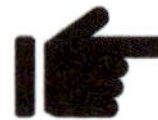

NOTE: Extra caution should be taken during this procedure to make the least amount of disturbance while dealing with differentiated C2C12 cells. Shear forces from pipetting the fluids into wells before the fixation step can induce contractions of myofibers and lift the cells off the plate.

1. Check the plate under the microscope for the presence of cells and the degree of differentiation. Note the notch on the plates to orient the plate. Different brands have different methods to orient the plate.
2. Remove the culture medium from the wells. This can be done by aspirating using pipette tips, a vacuum suction system, or by decanting into a tray. Decanting is easy and saves pipette tips and time. We will use decanting in this protocol.
3. Add 500 µl of DPBS(+) very gently along the side of each well. Rinse by gently swirling. Decant the solution into the waste collection tray. Repeat DPBS(+) rinse one more time and decant.

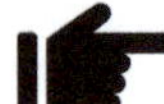

NOTE:

a. It is important to add the solutions very gently to the side of the wells. Shear forces generated during pipetting can lift the cells off the plate.

b. DPBS(+) must be used in procedures that require multiple rinses because DPBS without Ca^{++}/Mg^{++} can weaken cell attachment and lift the cells off the plate.

4. **Fixation and permeabilization**—Gently add 500 µl ice-cold (–20 °C) methanol per well and let stand for 10 min at room temperature. After incubation, decant methanol into the waste collection tray.
5. Perform two quick rinses using 500 µl DPBS(+) per well and decant into the waste collection tray.

6. **Blocking step**—Add 500 µl of 1% BSA blocking solution to each well. Incubate at room temperature for 10 min. BSA is a small sticky protein that will bind to any region on the plate where other proteins such as antibodies can bind. BSA coating prevents the nonspecific binding of antibodies and molecules, preventing nonspecific signals.
7. During the BSA incubation period, prepare the primary antibody reagent by diluting MF20 antibody 1:500 in antibody dilution buffer. If using antibodies from different vendors, follow the manufacturer's instructions for preparing the dilutions and incubation times.
8. After 10 min of blocking, decant the blocking solution into the waste collection tray.
9. **Detection step**—Add 250 µl primary antibody per well. Incubate at room temperature for 60 min. Alternatively, wrap the plate using parafilm and incubate overnight at 4 °C.

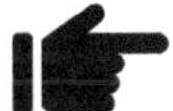

NOTE: Discuss the importance and relevance of proper experimental controls in research involving immunocytochemistry methods (antibody controls, positive controls, negative controls, etc.)

10. Prepare 1:500 dilution of the secondary antibody in the antibody dilution buffer. Green or red fluorescing secondary antibody may be used (see supply list).
11. Decant the primary antibody into the waste collection tray. Perform three quick rinses using 500 µl of DPBS(+) per well. Decant DPBS(+) into the waste collection tray.
12. Add 250 µl secondary antibody per well. Incubate the plate at room temperature for 60 min in the dark inside a drawer to prevent photobleaching. Alternatively, cover the plates with aluminum foil.
13. After incubation, decant the secondary antibody solution and perform three quick rinses with 500 µl of DPBS(+). Decant DPBS(+) into the waste collection tray.
14. **Counter staining step**—Perform counterstaining by adding 500 µl of DAPI nuclear stain per well. Incubate at room temperature for 10 min.
15. Decant the staining solution into the waste collection tray. Add 500 µl fresh DPBS(+) per well. Cells are ready for observation by fluorescence microscopy. Image the cells using phase contrast and fluorescence microscopy using filters for Alexa Fluor 488 (green) and DAPI (blue) (see sample image in Figure I 5.2). If using Alexa Fluor 568, use the red filter for actin stain.
16. If the plates are to be imaged at a later date, replace DPBS(+) with 500 µl of 0.1% sodium azide. Sodium azide prevents bacterial growth. Seal the plate with parafilm and store it in the fridge.

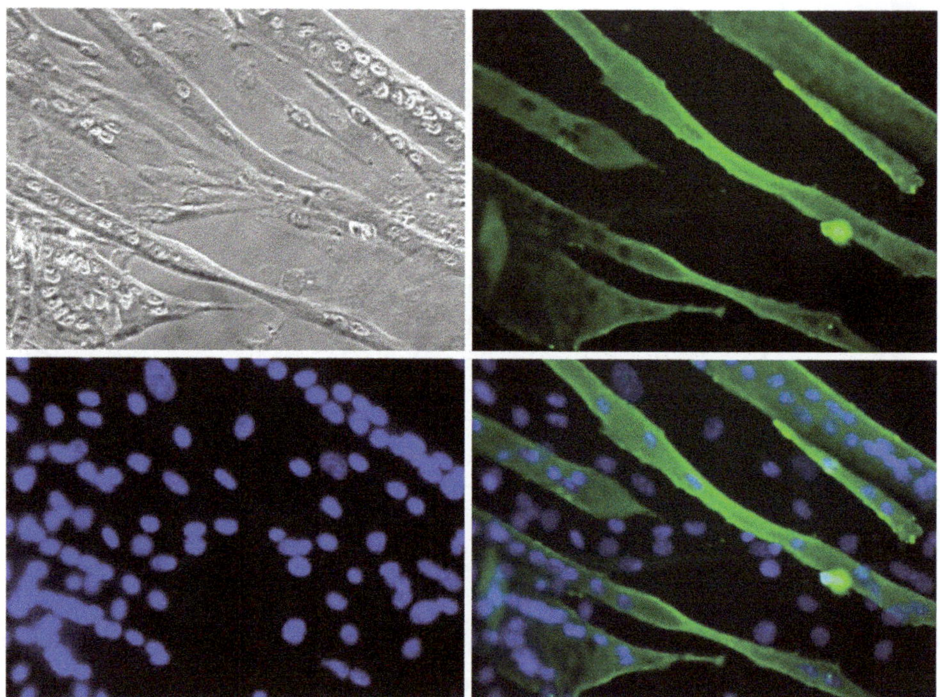

FIGURE I 5.2 Myosin heavy chain expression in differentiated C2C12 cells. The image panel represents a phase contrast image of myofibers (top left), myosin heavy chain expression in myofibers (green, top right), DAPI-stained nuclei (blue, bottom left), and myosin heavy chain and DAPI stain overlay (bottom right). Images were captured using a Zeiss Axiovert fluorescence microscope (400X magnification)

SUPPLY LIST—This list is for guidance only. Equivalent products may be used based on lab preferences.

Item	Vendor	Catalog #
C2C12 cells	ATCC	CRL-1772
4-well plate	VWR	62407-068
Methanol	VWR	JT9070-13
DPBS(+)	VWR	45000-430
Tween 20	VWR	95059-248
BSA, Fraction V (powder)	VWR	RLBSA50
*Anti myosin antibody (mouse IgG2b)	DSHB	MF20
*Alexa Fluor 488 Goat anti-Mouse IgG2b Cross-Adsorbed Secondary Antibody	Thermo Fisher	A-21141
*Alexa Fluor 568 Goat anti-Mouse IgG2b Cross-Adsorbed Secondary Antibody	Thermo Fisher	A-21144
DAPI	VWR	89139-118
Sodium azide	VWR	AA14314-22

* If you are using myosin primary antibody from a different vendor, use the appropriate secondary antibody.

Cell Proliferation Assay Using 5-Bromo-2'-Deoxyuridine

This procedure requires overnight incubation with the primary antibody.

What should you expect to learn in this lab?

1. A method to analyze cell proliferation
2. Methods of fixing and permeabilizing cells
3. Principles of immunocytochemistry
4. Fluorescence markers
5. Fluorescence microscopy and image analysis

Principle of BrdU assay: DNA is composed of four nucleotides—adenine, cytosine, guanine, and thymine. The 5-bromo-2'-deoxyuridine (BrdU) labeling reagent used in this procedure is a nucleotide analog that can replace thymine when incorporated into newly synthesized DNA in proliferating cells. Cell cultures are pulsed with BrdU for a brief period, typically 2–4 hours. However, depending on the experimental objective(s), cells can be incubated with BrdU from 60 min to 24 hours.

Supplies (see vendors and catalog numbers listed in the table at the end of this protocol)

1. Required PPE (lab coat, gloves, safety goggles) as required by the institution
2. One 4-well plate per student plated with 25,000 or 50,000 of 3T3 cells (or the desired cell type) a day prior to the procedure.
3. DPBS(+)—Dulbecco's phosphate buffered saline (Ca++/Mg++)
4. Fixative—Ice cold methanol
5. Blocking solution—1% BSA in DPBS(+)
6. Antibody dilution buffer (0.05% Tween-20 in DPBS(+))
7. 1.5 normal HCl prepared in water
8. BrdU labeling reagent
9. **Primary antibody**

   Option 1—Anti-BrdU antibody G3G4 (mouse) from Developmental Studies Hybridoma Bank

   Option 2—Alexa Fluor 488-conjugated anti-BrdU antibody (Cat # IIB5) from Santacruz

   Option 3—Anti-BrdU antibody from your preferred vendor

10. **Secondary antibody**—If you are using a G3G4 primary antibody, use an appropriate anti-mouse secondary antibody conjugated with the fluorescent molecule of choice. G3G4 is a mouse IgG1 antibody. We will use a goat anti-mouse IgG1 secondary antibody in this procedure (see supply list). If using a different primary antibody, use the appropriate secondary antibody.
    The anti-BrdU antibody from Santacruz listed above comes conjugated with Alexa Fluor 488. It is meant for direct immunofluorescence. Therefore, there is no need for a secondary antibody with this antibody.
11. 200 ng/ml DAPI nuclear stain prepared in DPBS(+).
12. 0.1% Sodium azide prepared in DPBS(+)

Procedure

This protocol explains the procedure for determining cell proliferation for cells cultured in 24-well plates. If a different-sized multi-well plate is used, cell numbers and reagent volumes should be adjusted accordingly. This procedure requires overnight incubation with the primary antibody.

1. Wear appropriate PPE as required by your institution (lab coat, gloves, safety goggles).
2. On the day of the procedure, add the BrdU labeling reagent at a ratio of 1:100 into the wells to be assayed. To do this, prepare a master mix of culture medium plus BrdU labeling reagent. For example, if you are assaying 10 wells in a 24-well plate, you require 5 ml of medium/BrdU mixture @ 500 µl per well. Prepare 6 ml mixture by adding 60 µl BrdU solution to 6 ml complete medium. Mix the contents.
3. Aspirate medium from the wells to be assayed. Add 500 µl of the BrdU mix to each well.
4. Transfer the plate to the incubator and incubate for 2–4 hours **or the time required** per the experimental protocol. The duration of BrdU incubation is determined by the proliferative rate of cells. Slow-growing cells may require longer incubation with BrdU. This should be established ahead of time.
5. After the BrdU incubation, discard the media from the wells. This can be done by aspirating using pipette tips, a vacuum suction system, or by decanting into a tray. Decanting is easy and saves pipette tips and time. We will use decanting in this protocol.
6. Perform a quick rinse using 500 µl DPBS(+) per well and discard. Repeat DPBS(+) rinse two more times and discard DPBS(+).
7. Fixation step—Add 500 µl ice-cold methanol per well. Incubate for 10 minutes at room temperature. Methanol fixes and permeabilizes the cells simultaneously.
8. After methanol fixation, decant methanol and perform two quick rinses using 500 µl DPBS(+) per well, and discard DPBS(+).
9. Add 500 µl of 1.5 normal HCl (prepared in water) per well. Incubate at room temperature for 20 min.

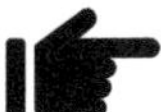

NOTE: The HCl incubation step helps nick and loosen the genomic DNA. This facilitates binding of primary antibody to the BrdU incorporated into the newly synthesized genomic DNA in cells that passed through the S phase of the cycle during the assay period.

The strength of HCl and the duration of treatment is crucial for the success of this procedure. High concentration and/or longer incubation times can destroy the genomic DNA. Lower concentration and/or shorter incubation will not produce enough nicks in DNA, restricting the ability of primary antibody to access and bind BrdU

10. Decant HCl after the incubation period.
11. Perform three quick rinses using 500 µl DPBS(+). After the final rinse, add 500 µl of DPBS(+) and incubate for 3 min at room temperature to dilute away any residual HCl. Decant DPBS(+).
12. Blocking step—Add 500 µl of 1% BSA blocking solution to each well. Incubate at room temperature for 10 min. BSA is a small sticky protein that will bind to any region on the plate where other proteins such as antibodies can bind. BSA coating prevents the nonspecific binding of antibodies and prevents nonspecific signals.
13. While step 12 is progressing, prepare the primary antibody. Make 1:100 dilution of anti-BrdU primary antibody (G3G4, DSHB) in antibody dilution buffer [DPBS(+)/0.05% Tween-20]. If using different primary antibodies, follow the manufacturer's protocol. If using the Santacruz antibody, make a 1:250 dilution of the antibody in the antibody dilution buffer
14. After the blocking step, decant the blocking solution.
15. Add 250 µl of primary antibody per well. Seal the plate using parafilm and incubate at 4 °C in the fridge overnight.
16. The following day, if the G3G4 primary antibody is used, prepare the secondary antibody by making a 1:500 dilution of Alexa Fluor 488 (green fluorescence) or Alexa Fluor 568 (red fluorescence) conjugated goat anti-Mouse IgG1 secondary antibody in antibody dilution buffer [DPBS(+)/0.05% Tween-20].

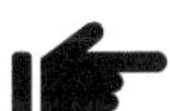

NOTE:

a. If a different primary antibody is used, use the appropriate secondary antibody and dilute it per the manufacturer's protocol.
b. If you are using the Santacruz antibody, a secondary antibody step is not required. Skip to step 19.

17. Decant the primary antibody. Perform three quick rinses using 500 µl DPBS(+).
18. Add 250 µl of fluorescence conjugated secondary antibody per well. Incubate at room temperature for 60 min in the dark (use aluminum foil to cover the plate or store it inside a drawer).

19. After incubation, decant secondary antibody (primary antibody if using Santacruz antibody).
20. Perform three quick rinses using 500 µl DPBS(+).
21. Add 500 µl 200 ng/ml DAPI in DPBS(+) or 0.5 µg/ml Hoechst in DPBS(+) staining solution. DAPI stain is preferred. Incubate for 10 min at room temperature.
22. Aspirate and discard the stain solution. Add 500 µl DPBS(+) per well. Cells are ready for observation by fluorescence microscopy. Cells that incorporated BrdU into their nuclei will show fluorescence signals in their nuclei (see sample images at the end of this protocol)
23. Calculate the ratio of cells that show BrdU incorporation (green or red fluorescence with Alexa Fluor 488 or 568, respectively) to all cells in the field of view (blue nuclei stained with DAPI or Hoechst). This can be done using ImageJ or similar software to automate the counting process. Green or red fluorescing nuclei represent the proportion of cells that incorporated the BrdU into their newly synthesized chromosomes during the duration of BrdU pulsing (see Figure I 6.1 at the end of this protocol).
24. If long-term storage of the BrdU plate is desired, aspirate DPBS(+) and add 0.1% sodium azide solution prepared in DPBS(+) to prevent bacterial growth. Seal the plate with parafilm and store at 4 °C.

SUPPLY LIST—This list is for guidance only. Equivalent products may be used based on lab preferences.

Item	Vendor	Catalog #
Cell type	Any cell type	
BrdU labeling reagent	Thermo Fisher	000103
6.0 N HCL	VWR	EM-HX0603M-6
Methanol	VWR	JT9070-13
DPBS(+)	VWR	45000-430
Tween 20	VWR	95059-248
BSA, Fraction V (powder)	VWR	RLBSA50
*Anti BrdU primary antibody (mouse IgG1)	DSHB	G3G4
*Alexa Fluor 488 Goat anti-Mouse IgG1 cross-adsorbed secondary antibody	Thermo Fisher	A-21121
*Alexa Fluor 568 Goat anti-Mouse IgG1 cross-adsorbed secondary antibody	Thermo Fisher	A-21124
**BrdU Antibody (IIB5) Alexa Fluor® 488	Santacruz	sc-32323 AF488
DAPI	VWR	89139-118
Sodium azide	VWR	AA14314-22

* If you are using anti-BrdU primary antibody from a different vendor, use the appropriate secondary antibody.

** The Santacruz ant-BrdU primary antibody is conjugated to Alexa Fluor-488 fluorescent molecule. Therefore, a secondary antibody step is not required.

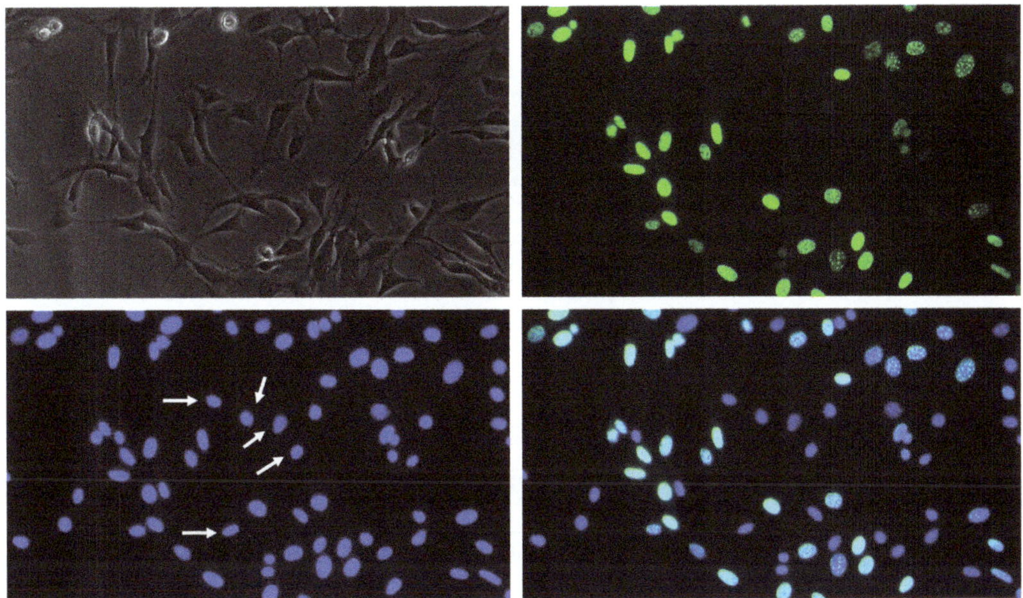

FIGURE I 6.1 Cell proliferation assay in 3T3 cells after 3 hr of BrdU labeling. Cells that incorporated BrdU into the newly synthesized genomic DNA as they passed through the S phase of the cell cycle during the 3 hr of BrdU labeling will exhibit green fluorescence in their nuclei. The images above represent the phase contrast image of 3T3 cells (top left), BrdU-labeled nuclei (green, top right), DAPI-stained nuclei (blue, bottom left), and overlay of BrdU and DAPI (bottom right). DAPI stains all nuclei in the field of view. BrdU is incorporated in a proportion of the cells. White arrows indicate examples of nuclei/cells that did not uptake BrdU during the assay period. Images were captured using a Zeiss Axiovert fluorescence microscope (200X magnification)

Independent Projects

Preparation for IPS

Serial Dilution for Seeding Specific Numbers of Cells on Small PDMS Pieces

Objectives

- ✓ Learn to perform serial dilution of cells.
- ✓ Determine optimal drop size of cell suspension for one square inch PDMS piece.
- ✓ Determine optimal cell density for the optimal drop size for one square inch PDMS piece so that the cells will be of reasonable confluency on day 5 to 7 after cell growth.
- ✓ Determine optimal time for cells to attach to PDMS before adding medium to cover the PDMS.
- ✓ Learn to image cells at different focal planes. The PDMS pieces may be of different thickness. You should learn to adjust the focal plane of the microscope objective to bring the cells into focus on top of the PDMS.

Overview

This procedure is intended to teach students the art of seeding cells on small pieces of a test substrate. Polydimethylsiloxane (PDMS) is used as the test substrate due to its versatility and ease of imaging cells. This can be applied to any other material, be it transparent or opaque, especially in the field of biomedical engineering, where biocompatibility of the substrate needs to be evaluated. This protocol will guide students through the process of ensuring that similar cell density is achieved on multiple PDMS pieces so that comparisons can be drawn at the end of the experiment.

Supplies

- 1" × 1" PDMS pieces
- 3T3 cells in 1.5 ml microcentrifuge tubes at 1×10^6 cells/ml (1000 cells/µl density) in complete medium
- Sterile 1.5 ml microcentrifuge tubes
- 60-mm tissue culture plates

- DMEM complete medium
- DPBS(+) or (–)

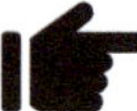

NOTE: This is a team project. While one group prepares for the serial dilution, the other group can perform step 2 and prepare for step 3.

Procedure

1. Serial dilution of cells: See details in Figure PI 1.1
   a. Take one 1.5 ml centrifuge tube containing 1 million cells per ml (1000 cell/µl) the instructor has provided you (tube #1). Place it in the microcentrifuge tube rack.
   b. Place five empty sterile 1.5 ml centrifuge tubes (marked #2 to #6) in the microcentrifuge tube rack and mark cell numbers per microliter (800, 400, 200, 100, 50) as shown in Figure PI 1.1.
   c. Add the specified volumes of DMEM complete medium to the respective tubes.
   d. Mix tube #1, containing one million cells per ml stock right before making the first dilution.
   e. Transfer 400 µl of cells suspension from tube #1 to tube #2, already containing 100 µl DMEM complete medium (see step c). This makes 500 µl cell suspension at 800 cells/µl.
   f. From here, you will be making 1:2 dilutions serially from tube 2 to 3, 3 to 4, 4 to 5, and 5 to 6 (hence the term "serial dilution"). Please make sure to mix the cell suspensions after each dilution to make a uniform cell suspension right before taking a sample and adding to the next tube.
   g. Now, you have a series of tubes containing cells at a density of 1000, 800, 400, 200, 100, and 50 cells per µl (note that the cell number is per µl, not per ml).

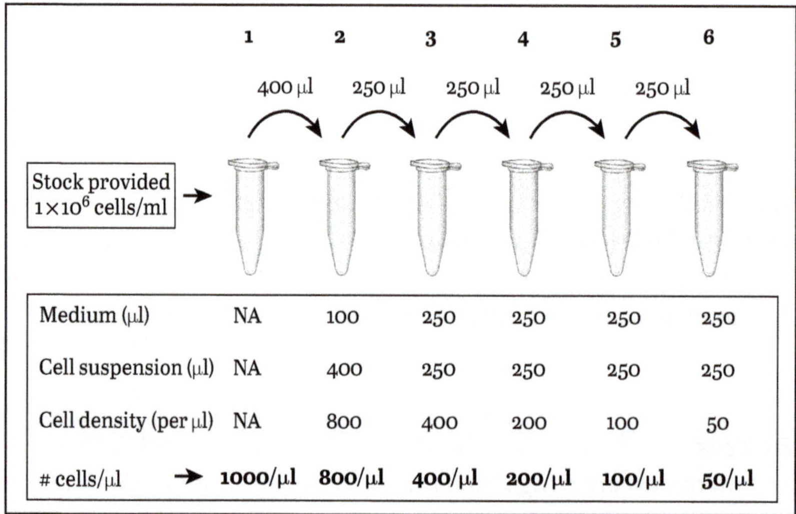

Medium (µl)	NA	100	250	250	250	250
Cell suspension (µl)	NA	400	250	250	250	250
Cell density (per µl)	NA	800	400	200	100	50
# cells/µl →	**1000/µl**	**800/µl**	**400/µl**	**200/µl**	**100/µl**	**50/µl**

FIGURE IP 1.1 Copyright © by Database Center for Life Science (DBCLS) (CC BY 3.0) at https://commons.wikimedia.org/wiki/File:Microtube2.png.

2. Determine optimal drop volume:

   a. Take enough PDMS pieces and place them in a 60-mm plate.
   b. Add different volumes of DPBS, ranging from 25 µl to 150 µl, in increments of 25 µl volumes, on to separate PDMS pieces.
   c. Determine which drop size is optimal so that it will not overflow while handling or transporting the PDMS pieces. At the same time the droplet should cover a large enough area on the PDMS piece that can hold a reasonable cell density on the PDMS surface. Note down the volume in your notebook. You will use this volume for seeding cells in stage 3 explained below.

3. Determine optimal cell density:

   a. Take enough PDMS pieces (6 pieces for 6 densities from stage 1) and place them in a 60-mm plate. You will be making drops of cell suspension for each serial dilution you prepared in stage 1 above. The volume of cells suspension is the optimal drop volume you determined in stage 2 above.
   b. Using a P200 pipette, seed the cells suspension from each serial dilution at the optimal drop volume you determined in step 2. For example, if you determined 50 µl to be the optimal drop size, seed 50 µl of cell suspension *from all dilutions* on 6 PDMS pieces placed in the 60-mm culture plate. If a 60-mm plate is not enough, you may use a 100-mm culture plate.
   c. Add 500 µl of DMEM complete medium to the 60 mm plate without disturbing the PDMS pieces. This will convert the 60 mm plate into a humidified chamber during the 2–3 hours of incubation. Humidification will prevent or minimize evaporation of the cell droplets.
   d. Close the lid and transfer the plate to the 37 °C incubator for about 15 minutes for the cells to settle to the PDMS surface. Image the cells in the droplets after the incubation period (time point zero).
   e. Imaging cells on PDMS surface is challenging. To image the cells after the 15-minute incubation, place the 60-mm plate on the microscope stage. Use the coarse adjustment to bring the 10x objective to touch the bottom of the plate.
   f. Move the microscope stage so that the center of the droplet you want to observe is brought above the 10x objective. While observing through the eye piece, gradually bring the objective down using the coarse adjustment, until the top surface of PDMS and cells come into focus.
   g. Identify the region with the most cell density. This is typically the center of the droplet. Take at least one representative image per drop. You must have an idea as to how trypsinized cells should look under the phase contrast (rounded and refractile). Please do not confuse random features within the PDMS for cells.
   h. After imaging is complete, return the 60-mm plate to the incubator for up to 2 to 3 hours. Check for cell attachment every 45 to 60 minutes. Attachment will be evident when a proportion of the cells show spreading. They will also resist rolling around when the drop is shaken. Take images for each density. Discard the plates after 3 hours of incubation and imaging.
   i. Based on your observations, determine which droplet has the optimal cell density. This determination should be based on the space the cells occupy in the droplet that would

permit good cell proliferation without being too confluent in 5–7 days. This, in turn, is based on your experience with cell dynamics with the PDL independent project you have been doing since early in the term.

j. Note all of the observations in your lab notebook. You will use the information from this experiment in a separate independent project entitled **Surface coating of small PDMS pieces, Cell seeding, and Cell growth**.

Biocompatibility and Toxicity Testing

Objectives

- ✓ Learn how to set up experiments.
- ✓ Learn sterilization protocols.
- ✓ Identify biocompatibility and toxicity of test materials to 3T3 cells.

Supplies

- 12-well tissue culture treated plates
- Test materials (see Table PI 2.1)
- NIH/3T3 cells at 50,000 cells/ml in DMEM complete medium in a 50 ml tube
- Forceps, isopropyl alcohol, and DPBS(–) in 15-ml tubes
- UV sterilization box

TABLE PI 2.1 Test Materials

Item	Your hypothesis	
	Biocompatible	**Toxic**
Stainless steel ring		
Nylon ring		
Copper ring		
Brass ring		
Super glue		
Gorilla glue		
Loctite super glue		
Liquid band aid		
Sylgard 184 silicone elastomer base		

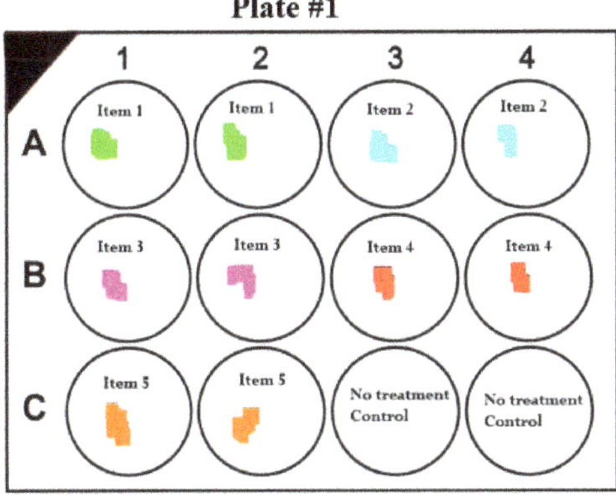

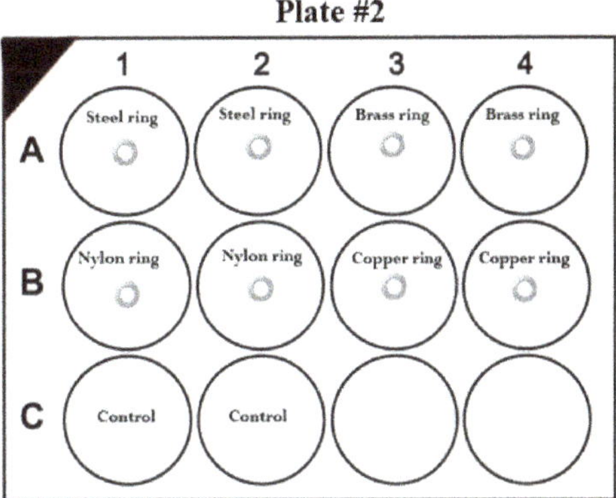

FIGURE PI 2.1

Procedure

1. Bring two 12-well Bring two 12-well tissue-culture-treated plates per team inside the culture hood. Check the orientation of the wells by identifying the corner notch and wells A1–A4 through C1–C4. The corner notch helps orient the plate. Different brands of plates have different methods for orienting the plate.
2. Mark duplicate wells for each test material, as shown in Figure PI 2.1.
3. **Plate #1:** Using a P200 pipette tip, take one drop (about 10 μl) of each test material, and place it slightly to the left or right of the midline of the corresponding wells, as marked in Figure PI 2.1. For some of the test materials, you may have to squeeze the tube and use the pipette tip to scoop up a similar sized drop of the material. *Use new pipette tip for each test material.* Leave the control wells empty.
4. After all test materials have been dispensed, move the plate to one side or the far corner of the hood away from you. Keep the lid of plate #1 open inside the hood for 15 minutes to allow it to vent. Ensure that nothing passes above the open wells.
5. **Plate #2:** While plate #1 is venting, prepare plate #2. Sterilize the forceps by immersing it in isopropyl alcohol in a 15-ml tube for 5 minutes. After sterilization, perform two sequential rinses by dipping the forceps in DPBS (–) in 15-ml tubes #1 and #2 respectively. You can place the forceps in a clean, sterile 100-mm plate to dry, if needed.
6. Using the sterile forceps, pick up the metal and nylon rings and place them in the center of the corresponding wells, as shown in Figure PI 2.1. There is no need to sterilize the forceps between the different rings. Close the lid.
7. After both plates are ready, close the lids and bring them to the UV sterilization box. Sterilize the plates and their contents (with the lid closed) by applying UV light for 20 minutes in the "all" position for UV application from the top and bottom of the plates.
8. After sterilization, bring the plates inside the culture hood. *Do not open the lid outside the hood.*
9. Mix the 3T3 cells (50,000/ml) in the 50-ml tube by inverting the tube a few times.
10. Using a P1000 micropipette, add 1 ml cell suspension to each well, including control wells.
11. Transfer the plates to the incubator and allow 15 to 20 minutes for the cells to settle to the bottom.
12. After the 15–20-minute incubation, check every well under the microscope to ensure that all wells have been seeded with cells and their densities are about equal. At this time, every well should look about the same. Image the two "control" wells. *It is best to image in the center of the well.* This is your baseline at time point 0. You will use these images to compare against images taken later to determine the effect of the test materials on 3T3 cells.
13. **Day 3/4:** Observe each well under the microscope. For each well, take at least one representative image of cells at the edge of the test material and its adjacent region. Take another image slightly away from the test material. Depending on your preference, you may image using the 5x and/or 10x objective (make sure to use the appropriate phase ring). You may take more images, as necessary. Note your observations for each test material in your lab notebook. Specifically, check for the following:

  i. Cells are healthy, attached, spreading, and proliferating well (similar to the control).
  ii. Cells are dead, shriveled, and floating, with no proliferation.
  iii. Cells look unhealthy and barely surviving, with minimal or no proliferation.
  iv. Is there a "dead zone" around the test material with normal cell growth in other areas?
  v. Note any other observations or variations.

14. Tabulate and interpret your results. Explain why some materials are biocompatible, why some are toxic, and why some are in-between. Explain why this testing method is important in the field of biomedical engineering.
15. Try to research the chemical composition of the test materials and hypothesize the reason for the results to the best of your abilities.

TABLE PI 2.2 Supply List: Vendors and Catalog Numbers

Item	Vendor	Cat #
12-well tissue culture treated plate	Any brand	Multiple
NIH/3T3 cells	ATCC	CRL-1658
Stainless steel ring (M2.5 stainless steel washers, 200 per pack)	Amazon.com	N/A
Nylon ring (M2.5 plastic nylon washers, 100 per pack)	Amazon.com	N/A
Copper ring (M2.5 copper washers, 100 per pack)	Amazon.com	N/A
Brass ring (M2.5 brass washers, 300 per pack)	Amazon.com	N/A
Super glue	Store bought	N/A
Gorilla glue	Store bought	N/A
Loctite super glue	Store bought	N/A
Liquid band aid	Store bought	N/A
SYLGARD 184 Silicone Elastomer Kit	Dow	N/A

Contact Angle Measurement

Objectives

To identify the "wettability" of various surfaces by determining the contact angle of water droplets placed on the surfaces.

1. Understand the principle of contact angles produced by water droplets on various surfaces.
2. Determine the hydrophilicity and hydrophobicity of materials based on contact angle measurements.
3. Explore methods to modify the wettability of substrates.

Supplies

1. Tissue culture-treated surface of a 60 mm culture plate with the rim removed for easy imaging of the water droplets.
2. The surface of a 60 mm petri dish (untreated and NOT suited for mammalian cell culture) with the rim removed for easy imaging of the water droplets.
3. Glass microscope slides
4. PDMS pieces (3" × 1")
5. Water (with blue food color added for contrast for better imaging) in 1.5 ml tubes
6. Clean white printer paper
7. 70% isopropyl alcohol in a spray bottle
8. Plasma cleaner
9. Micropipette, pipette tips, forceps, paper towel

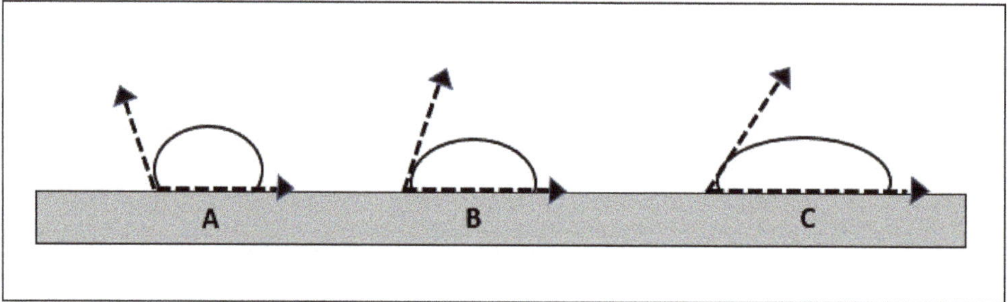

FIGURE PI 3.1

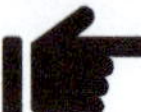

NOTE: Images should be taken at the same level as the surface of the water droplets to obtain good contact angle measurements. Other angles will give you erratic measurements.

1. This is a team project. You may use your own smartphones to image the droplets placed on the different surfaces.
2. This work is performed outside the hood since the project does not require sterile conditions.
3. Each team will pick up the necessary items from the list above and bring them to the work area.
4. Fold the white printer paper in half. One half forms the base to place the test materials for contact angle measurements and the other half becomes the background to help with imaging.
5. Bring the PDMS pieces to the sink. Spray the pieces with 70% isopropyl alcohol, rinse in cold running tap water, and wipe dry with paper towels. Bring the pieces back to the work area. Place the PDMS pieces on the folded white paper.
6. Place items 1 and 2 from the list above (60 mm plates without rims) and the glass slide (item 3) on the folded white paper.
7. Set the P-200 pipette to 25 µl. Make three droplets of the blue-colored water side by side in a straight line on the surfaces of the test materials closer to the edge. The droplets should be placed with enough distance between the droplets so that they do not touch each other. However, they should be close enough so that you can get all three droplets in one image.
8. Using your smartphone, take images of each droplet separately or all three droplets in one image.

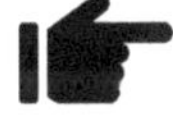

NOTE 1: To make the droplets, hold the micropipette vertically and the pipette tip close to the surface. Rest the elbow on the surface of the bench and use the other hand to steady the pipette tip. Make the droplet gently by allowing the tip to touch the growing droplet as you pipette the fluid. This method makes better droplets compared to holding the pipette in a slanted position.

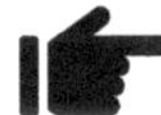

NOTE 2: If you have trouble getting sharp focus with your camera, hold another object such as a pipette tip right above the droplet so that the camera is able to maintain the focus.

---

9. After imaging the droplets on untreated PDMS pieces, rinse the PDMS pieces under running tap water and wipe dry with a paper towel.
10. Subject the PDMS piece(s) to plasma treatment using the optimal settings for the plasma oxygen cleaner in the lab. This is typically done for 30 seconds to 2 minutes. Make sure to follow the specific instructions provided by your course instructor.

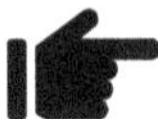

NOTE 3: Plasma treatment occurs only on the surfaces that are exposed to oxygen plasma. Therefore, it is important to keep track of the treated surface. After the treatment, handle the PDMS only with a pair of clean forceps.

---

11. Bring the plasma-treated PDMS to the workbench. Place it on the folded white paper. Make only one droplet on the plasma-treated surface. If the plasma treatment has worked well, the effect will be dramatic. If you want to make three measurements, treat different PDMS pieces. Image the droplets.
12. Perform image analysis on the imaged droplets. The contact angle is the angle formed by the intersection of the baseline and the tangent that touches the curvature of the drop as shown in the image above (Figure PI 3.1).
13. Image analysis can be done in multiple ways:

    a. The old-fashioned way—print out the images and use a protractor to measure the contact angle as indicated in the image above
    b. Any protractor tool available online
    c. Use the "angle" feature in ImageJ
    d. Use the automated feature in ImageJ

14. Discuss the importance of contact angle measurements in your lab report. Determine which of the surfaces are hydrophilic, hydrophobic, super hydrophilic, or super hydrophobic as applicable.
15. Discuss other ways to modify surface properties and how this can be applied to improve cell attachment or to prevent cell attachment to the materials(s).

Coating of Cell Culture Surfaces

Objectives

- ✓ Explore the effect of coating of culture surfaces on cell attachment, growth, and proliferation.
- ✓ Understand the mechanics of surface coating.
- ✓ Learn how to prepare coating materials in proper solvents at the optimal concentrations.
- ✓ Learn about the conditions when rinsing and drying of coated surface is necessary.
- ✓ Learn cell imaging.

Supplies

- 24-well non-tissue culture plates (one per team)
- 35-mm tissue-culture-treated plate (one per team)
- sterile water
- 3T3 cells at 20,000 cells/ml in 10% FBS complete medium in a 15-ml tube
- substrate for coating the wells
    - a. bovine collagen, type I (PureCol EZ Gel)—100 µg/ml in sterile water
    - b. gelatin from porcine skin— 2 mg/ml in sterile water
    - c. Poly-D-lysine solution—50 µg/ml in sterile water
    - d. Poly-L-ornithine solution—50 µg/ml in sterile water
    - e. Dopamine hydrochloride solution—2 mg/ml in 10 mM Tris-HCl, pH 8.5 and filter sterilized (prepared fresh and filter-sterilized right before the coating procedure)
    - f. Poly(2-hydroxyethyl methacrylate) (Poly-HEMA)—70 mg/ml in 200 proof ethanol

---

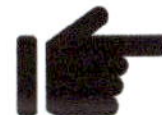

NOTE: You should have researched the properties of the coating materials by now and developed an idea about the solvents used for each coating, optimal concentrations, and the duration of coating. The instructor may provide preprepared coating solutions or students may prepare the coating solution from concentrated stocks.

---

1. Use one 24-well **non-tissue culture plate** per team. Bring the plate inside the culture hood. Check the orientation of the wells by identifying the corner notch and wells A1–A6 through D1–D6. The corner notch helps orient the plate (different brands of plates may have different notch patterns).
2. Team members should decide how to divide the labor for this project. Mark duplicate wells for each coating material. Two wells in the plate will be used as non-coated control wells (negative control) (Figure PI 4.1).

3. Add 500 µl of each coating solution to the corresponding wells. Please remember that the **non-tissue culture treated** wells are hydrophobic. Therefore, lower volume of coating substrate may not wet the wells properly. If 500 µl volume is inadequate to cover the surface, add enough coating solution to cover the well surface as necessary.
4. Incubate the plate for 1 hour at room temperature inside the biosafety cabinet.
5. After the incubation period, aspirate and discard the coating solutions from the wells.
6. Gently add 500 µl of sterile water to the wells, rinse the plate gently, aspirate, and discard the contents from the wells.
7. Move the plate to one side of the biosafety cabinet. With the lid open, air dry the plate inside the biosafety cabinet for 15–20 minutes or until the wells are completely dry. The air circulation inside the hood enhances drying. Take care not to pass anything above the plate while the lid is open.
8. Mix the cells in the 15-ml tube using a serological pipette or by inverting the tube a few times..
9. Using a P-1000 pipette, add 2 ml of the cell suspension to the 35 mm tissue culture treated plate (positive control plate, 40,000 cells total).
10. Add 500-µl cell suspension to each well in the coated wells and the control (non-coated) wells (10,000 cells per well).
11. Transfer the plate to the 37 °C incubator and incubate for 15–20 minutes for cells to settle to the bottom.
12. Check the 35-mm positive control plate and all the wells in the 24-well plate for the presence of cells. All wells in the 24-well plate should have similar densities at this point.
13. Image the 35-mm plate (two images) and at least two wells of the 24-well plate. Image the cells in the center of the well for good contrast. This is time point zero reference. Return the plate to the incubator.
14. Image all wells in the 24-well plate and positive control plate on days 4 and 7.
15. Analyze, and quantify your results.

    a. What was the purpose of using a **non-tissue culture treated plate** for this experiment?
    b. Did you observe discernible differences in the morphology of the cells for the different treatments? If yes, explain the reason(s) for the differences and relate it to the chemical property of the coating materials.
    c. Did you observe differences in the rate of proliferation between different coatings? If yes, how can you quantify the differences?
    d. Interpret your results and explain how each coating material impacted cell morphology and proliferation.

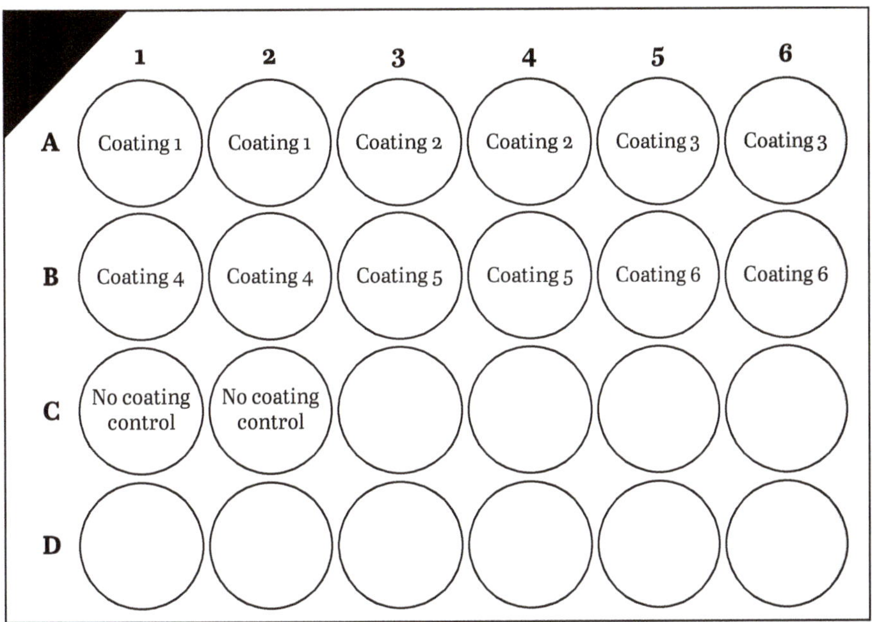

FIGURE PI 4.1

TABLE PI 3.1 Supply List: Vendors and Catalog Numbers

Item	Vendor	Catalog #
NIH/3T3 cells	ATCC	CRL-1658
Bovine collagen, type I (PureCol EZ Gel)	Advanced Biomatrix	5074-35ML
Gelatin from porcine skin	Millipore Sigma	G1890-100G
Poly-D-Lysine solution	ThermoFisher	A3890401
Poly-L-Ornithine powder	Advanced Biomatrix	5172
Dopamine hydrochloride	Millipore Sigma	H8502-25G
Poly(2-hydroxyethyl methacrylate) (Poly-HEMA)	Millipore Sigma	P3932-10G
24-well non-tissue culture plate	Any brand	Multiple
35-mm tissue-culture-treated plate	Any brand	Multiple
Tris-HCl (1M), pH 8.5. 1000 mL, Sterile	Teknova	T1085

Determining Population Doubling Level of Cells

Objectives

- ✓ Understand cell counting.
- ✓ Learn the difference between cell passaging and cell doubling.
- ✓ Understand factors that affect cell proliferation.
- ✓ Calculate cell population doubling time.

The Effect of FBS Concentration on Cell Proliferation

This is an independent team project. Each student will manage one culture plate throughout this independent project. The project is intended to help students understand the effect of the concentration of fetal bovine serum (FBS) on the PDL of 3T3 cells over the duration of the study. Team members will decide who will manage which FBS concentration. The cells will be subcultured once a week. The project will run for 4–5 weeks for a total of 4–5 passages.

Through this exercise you will gain expertise in the art of subculturing, media preparation, sterile culture technique, cell counting, microscopic evaluation of cells, cell imaging and determining population doubling level, cumulative PDL, and time taken by the cells (in hours) to undergo one cell division.

Reagents and Supplies

- Prepare your own complete media. Prepare 50 ml of complete media at a time in 50-ml tubes. Label them with your name or initials and date of media preparation. Save your tube in your assigned rack in the fridge. Prepare fresh complete media, as needed.
- Complete culture media composition—DMEM supplemented with 10% or 8% FBS, 1x Glutamax and 1x Penn/strep

Procedure

In this exercise, teams will compare the growth and proliferation of NIH/3T3 cells in different concentrations of fetal bovine serum (10% and 8%) over a period of 4–5 weeks and, in turn, its effect on Population Doubling Level (PDL):

1. *Check the culture plate under the microscope to ensure that the culture is not contaminated.* Check the color, consistency, and clarity of culture medium. Write your observations in your lab notebook. Take an image of the cells using the 10X objective. Bring the culture plate into the hood.
2. Trypsinize the cells using the protocol you have been following so far. Transfer the cell suspension to a 15-ml centrifuge tube.
3. Check the plate to ensure significant numbers of cells are not left on the plate (see the Troubleshooting box below).
4. Use a sample of suspension to determine the cell count. Follow the cell counting protocol to determine the total cell count.
5. Place the 15-ml conical tube in the centrifuge and spin at 200 g to 250 g for 5–10 minutes.
6. While the cells are pelleting, count the cells in the four corner squares of the hemocytometer. Calculate cell count per ml and total cell count in the tube. Use dilution factor, if applicable.
7. After centrifugation, carefully aspirate the supernatant and resuspend the cell pellet in an appropriate volume of complete media to obtain 1×10^6 cells/ml (1,000 cells/µl).
8. Mix the cells in the tube to break up the pellet and to ensure uniform cell distribution.
9. Prepare fresh tissue culture plates for each FBS concentration. Mark the plate with the name of the cells, passage number, date of passage, FBS % and your initials. Add 10 ml of complete media to the plates.
10. Plate the following cell numbers for each FBS concentration in the corresponding plate:
    a. 100,000 cells (100 µl) from the 10% FBS plate
    b. 125,000 cells (125 µl) from the 8% FBS plate
11. Check the new culture plate under the microscope. Take an image for reference. Transfer the plate to the incubator.
12. From this point forward, you will subculture these cells *once a week*. Plate the cell numbers indicated in step 10 every time you subculture the cells until the endpoint for this project.
13. Keep note of the total cell count and the number of days intervening between subcultures to determine the PDL, cumulative PDL (cPDL), and average PDL time (in hours; see Table IP 1.1).
14. Calculate the PDL, using the formula below. From the data, calculate the cumulative PDL and the number of hours for your 3T3 cells to go through one round of replication (see Table IP 1.1).

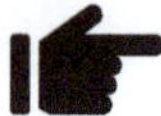

NOTE: PDL = 3.32 [log (total viable cells at harvest/total viable cells at seeding)]

---

15. Create a spreadsheet, as shown in Table IP 1.1. This allows you to keep track of the population doubling time more effectively. Plug in the formula for number of days, PDL, and cPDL calculations as well as for average PDL time. You may also use the PDL spreadsheet template posted on the course site.

TABLE IP 1.1 Sample Data Sheet for PDL Study

Day of plating	Day of subculture	Days in culture	Cells seeded on day of plating	Today's yield	PDL	Cumulative PDL	Average PDL time (hours)
1/4/2018	1/7/2018	3	100,000	480,000	2.26	2.26	31.8
1/7/2018	1/13/2018	6	100,000	2,440,000	4.61	6.87	31.2
1/13/2018	1/19/2018	6	100,000	3,050,000	4.93	11.80	29.2
1/19/2018	1/25/2018	6	100,000	2,930,000	4.81	16.68	29.6
1/25/2018	1/31/2018	6	100,000	3,128,000	4.97	21.64	29.0
1/31/2018	2/6/2018	6	100,000	3,114,000	4.96	26.60	29.0

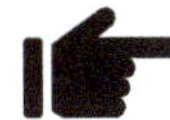

NOTE: If the yield of cells is too high or too low after 7 days in culture, you may adjust the seeding density for the specific treatment. However, make sure to note those changes in the spreadsheet.

Analysis

- Did you observe differences in cell proliferation between the two FBS treatments?
- Are the differences statistically significant?
- Present your results graphically.
- Explain and discuss your results in your lab report. Base your discussion on published literature.

TROUBLESHOOTING: If large patches of cells still remain on the plate after step 3, perform the following steps:

a. Rinse the plate once *very gently* with DPBS(−).
b. Repeat trypsinization per regular protocol, with 3 ml of trypsin.
c. Check the plate under the microscope to monitor the degree of trypsinization.
d. After trypsinization, add 2 ml of complete medium, for a total volume of 5 ml. Pipette vigorously to release the cells from the plate.
e. Collect 5 ml of cell suspension, and pool it with the cell suspension already in the 15 ml tube from first isolation.

TABLE IP 1.2 Supply List: Vendors and Catalog Numbers

Item	Vendor	Catalog #
NIH/3T3 cells	ATCC	CRL-1658
100 mm × 20 mm Tissue Culture Treated Dishes With Grip Ring	Chemglass	CLS-1805-152
DMEM media (with 4.5 g/L glucose and sodium pyruvate, without L-glutamine)	VWR	45000-316
Fetal bovine serum	Your choice	
Glutamax supplement (100x)	Thermo Fisher	35050061
Penicillin: Streptomycin solution 100x, Corning	VWR	45000-652
DPBS(−)	VWR	45000-434
Four-Chip Disposable Hemocytometer, four chambers per chip	VWR	102966-632
Double Neubauer Chamber With Two Cover glasses	VWR	102094-780

Effect of Growth Factor

Objectives

- ✓ Understand cell counting.
- ✓ Learn the difference between cell passaging and cell doubling.
- ✓ Understand the factors that affect cell proliferation (bFGF).
- ✓ Calculate cell population doubling time.

The Effect of Growth Factor Concentration on Cell Proliferation

This is an independent team project. Each student will manage two culture plates, one plate cultured under the normal condition (control culture) and the second plate supplemented with either 4 ng/ml bFGF or 10 ng/ml bFGF. Team members will decide who will manage which bFGF concentration. The cells will be subcultured twice a week. The project will run for 3 weeks for a total of 6 passages for each culture.

Through this exercise you will gain expertise in the art of subculturing, media preparation, sterile culture technique, cell counting, microscopic evaluation of cells, cell imaging and determining population doubling level, cumulative PDL, and time taken by the cells (in hours) to undergo one cell division.

Reagents and Supplies

- Prepare your own complete media. Prepare 50 ml of complete media at a time in 50-ml tubes. Label the tube with your name or initials and date of media preparation. Save your tube in your assigned rack in the fridge. Prepare fresh complete media, as needed.
- Complete culture media composition—DMEM supplemented with 10% FBS, 1x Glutamax and 1x Penn/strep
- bFGF—Each team will get their own vial of bFGF prepared at 10 µg/ml. Please label the aliquot and store it in the bFGF box in the −20°C freezer. The bFGF should be added to the cultures only at the time of subculturing and cell seeding. Outside the freezer, keep the bFGF vial on ice at all times. Minimize freeze–thaw cycles.

Procedure

In this exercise, teams will compare the growth and proliferation of NIH/3T3 cells in different concentrations of basic fibroblast growth factor over a period of 3 weeks. Students are provided with a plate of NIH/3T3 cells at the beginning of this independent project. You should carry the cells forward on your own. If a mishap happens during the project, you may borrow cells from the same treatment (with or without bFGF) from other students in your lab section:

1. *Check the culture plate under the microscope to ensure that the culture is not contaminated.* Check the color, consistency, and clarity of culture medium. Write your observations in your lab notebook. Take an image using 10x objective. Bring the culture plate into the hood.
2. Trypsinize the cells using the protocol you have been following so far. Transfer the cell suspension to a 15-ml centrifuge tube.
3. Check the plate to ensure significant numbers of cells are not left on the plate (see the Troubleshooting box below).
4. Use a sample of suspension to determine the cell count. Follow the cell counting protocol to determine the total cell count.
5. Place the 15-ml conical tube in the centrifuge and spin at 200 g to 250 g for 5–10 minutes.
6. While the cells are pelleting, count the cells in the four corner squares of the hemocytometer. Calculate cell count per ml and total cell count in the tube. Use dilution factor, if applicable.
7. After centrifugation, carefully aspirate the supernatant and resuspend the cell pellet in an appropriate volume of complete media to obtain 1×10^6 cells/ml (1,000 cells/µl).
8. Mix the cells in the tube to break up the pellet and to ensure uniform cell distribution.
9. Prepare two 100-mm fresh tissue culture plates for each student—one for cells without bFGF supplementation and one for cells with bFGF supplementation. Mark the plates with all the necessary details. Add 9.5 ml of complete medium to the plates.
10. Add 500,000 cells (500 µl cell suspension) to each plate.
11. To the bFGF plate, add the necessary amount of bFGF. Since you will be adding quite a small amount of the growth factor (10 microliters or less), make sure that you deliver the growth factor into the culture medium by touching the tip of the pipette into the medium. Repeat pipetting up and down with the same pipette tip a few times to ensure that all the growth factor is delivered into the medium.
12. Mix the cells in both plates by gently tilting them forward, backward, and sideways.
13. Check the plates under the microscope. Take images and transfer the plate to the incubator.
14. From this point forward, you will subculture these cells *twice a week*. For every subculture, plate the cell numbers indicated in step 10. Continue until the endpoint of this project.
15. Create a spreadsheet with details, as shown in Table IP 2.1. Alternatively, you may use the Excel sheet posted on the course site by the instructor. Update the spreadsheet every time you passage the cells. You will use these details to determine the PDL, cumulative PDL (cPDL), and the average time (hours) it takes for the cells to replicate once.
16. Compare and contrast the growth rate of cells for the growth factor treatment against no growth factor control using proper statistical analysis.

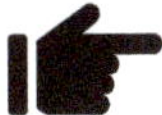

NOTE: PDL = 3.32 [log (total viable cells at harvest/total viable cells at seeding)]

TABLE IP 2.1 Sample data sheet for PDL study

Day of plating	Day of subculture	Days in culture	Cells seeded on day of plating	Today's yield	PDL	Cumulative PDL	Average PDL time (hours)
1/4/2018	1/7/2018	3	100,000	480,000	2.26	2.26	31.8
1/7/2018	1/13/2018	6	100,000	2,440,000	4.61	6.87	31.2
1/13/2018	1/19/2018	6	100,000	3,050,000	4.93	11.80	29.2
1/19/2018	1/25/2018	6	100,000	2,930,000	4.81	16.68	29.6
1/25/2018	1/31/2018	6	100,000	3,128,000	4.97	21.64	29.0
1/31/2018	2/6/2018	6	100,000	3,114,000	4.96	26.60	29.0

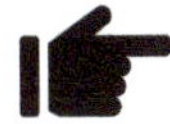

NOTE: If the yield of cells is too high or low in your treatment(s), you may adjust the seeding density for the specific treatment. Make sure to note those changes in the spreadsheet and explain the reasoning for the changes in your lab notebook.

TROUBLESHOOTING: If large patches of cells still remain on the plate after step 3, perform the following steps:

a. Rinse the plate once *very gently* with DPBS(−).
b. Repeat trypsinization per regular protocol, with 3 ml of trypsin.
c. Check the plate under the microscope to monitor the degree of trypsinization.
d. After trypsinization, add 2 ml of complete medium for a total volume of 5 ml. Pipette vigorously to release the cells from the plate.
e. Collect 5 ml of cell suspension and pool this with the cell suspension already in the 15-ml tube from first isolation.

TABLE IP 2.2 Supply List: Vendors and Catalog Numbers

Item	Vendor	Catalog #
NIH/3T3 cells	ATCC	CRL-1658
Basic fibroblast growth factor (bFGF)	Prospec	CYT-557
100 mm × 20 mm Tissue Culture Treated Dishes With Grip Ring	Chemglass	CLS-1805-152
DMEM media (with 4.5 g/L glucose and sodium pyruvate, without L-glutamine)	VWR	45000-316
Fetal bovine serum	Lab choice	Multiple
Glutamax supplement (100x)	Thermo Fisher	35050061
Penicillin: Streptomycin solution 100x, Corning	VWR	45000-652
DPBS(−)	VWR	45000-434
Four-Chip Disposable Hemocytometer, four chambers per chip	VWR	102966-632
Double Neubauer Chamber With Two Cover glasses	VWR	102094-780

Effect of Sodium Butyrate

Objectives

- ✓ Understand cell counting.
- ✓ Learn the difference between cell passaging and cell doubling.
- ✓ Understand factors that affect cell proliferation.
- ✓ Calculate cell population doubling time.

The Effect of Sodium Butyrate Concentration on Cell Proliferation

This project runs for the whole term (4–5 weeks). Through this exercise you will gain expertise in the art of subculturing, media preparation, sterile culture technique, cell counting, microscopic evaluation of cells, cell imaging and determining population doubling level, cumulative PDL, and time taken by the cells (in hours) to undergo one cell division.

Reagents and Supplies

- Prepare your own complete media. Prepare 50 ml of complete media at a time in 50-ml tubes. Label them with your name or initials and date of media preparation. Save your tube in your assigned rack in the fridge. Prepare fresh complete media, as needed.
- Complete culture media composition—DMEM supplemented with 10% FBS, 1x Glutamax and 1x Penn/strep
- Sodium butyrate—Students should read the literature to understand the effect of sodium butyrate on cell proliferation. Each team will get a tube of 1 M sodium butyrate. Please label the tube and store it in a rack in the fridge. The team should plan to use a range of sodium butyrate concentrations, starting week 3 of the project. **Sodium butyrate should be added to the cultures only at the time of subculturing and cell seeding.**

Procedure

In this exercise, teams will compare the growth and proliferation of NIH/3T3 cells in the presence of sodium butyrate over a period of 4–5 weeks. Students are provided with a plate of NIH/3T3 cells at the beginning of this independent project. You should carry the cells forward on your own. If a mishap happens during the project, you may borrow cells from other students in your lab section:

1. *Check the culture plate under the microscope to ensure that the culture is not contaminated.* Check the color, consistency, and clarity of culture medium. Write your observations in your lab notebook. Take an image using 10x objective. Bring the culture plate into the hood.
2. Trypsinize the cells using the protocol you have been following so far. Transfer the cell suspension to a 15-ml centrifuge tube.
3. Check the plate to ensure significant numbers of cells are not left on the plate (see the following Troubleshooting box).
4. Use a sample of suspension to determine the cell count. Follow the cell counting protocol to determine the total cell count.
5. Place the 15-ml conical tube in the centrifuge and spin at 200 g to 250 g for 5–10 minutes.
6. While the cells are pelleting, count the cells in the four corner squares of the hemocytometer. Calculate cell count per ml and total cell count in the tube. Use dilution factor, if applicable.
7. After centrifugation, carefully aspirate the supernatant and resuspend the cell pellet in an appropriate volume of complete media to obtain 1×10^6 cells/ml (1,000 cells/µl).
8. Mix the cells in the tube to break up the pellet and to ensure uniform cell distribution.
9. Prepare fresh tissue culture plates for this experiment. Mark the plate with the name of the cells, passage number, date of passage, and your initials. Add 10 ml of complete media to the plates.
10. Add 100,000 cells (100 µl) to the 10 ml medium in the plate.
11. Mix the cells in the plate(s) by gently tilting it forward, backward, and sideways.
12. Check the plates under the microscope. Take an image for reference. Transfer the plate to the incubator.
13. You will subculture this plate next week and prepare two plates per student - one control plate (no sodium butyrate) and one sodium butyrate treatment per student (see step 15 below).
14. From this point forward, you will subculture these cells *once a week*, for 4–5 weeks.
15. In the meantime, team members should decide the concentrations of sodium butyrate each student is going to manage. The suggested final concentrations for sodium butyrate are 500 µM, 1 mM, and 2.5 mM. Each student will continue with two culture plates—one control plate (no sodium butyrate) and a second plate with one of the sodium butyrate concentrations with cell densities indicated below. Between the team members, all suggested concentrations should be covered.

    a. seeding density for control plates
    100,000 cells per 100-mm plate—one plate per student

    b. seeding density for sodium butyrate plates.
    500 µM sodium butyrate—500,000 cells per 100-mm plate, one plate per student
    1 mM sodium butyrate—1 million cells per 100-mm plate, one plate per student
    2.5 mM sodium butyrate—1 million cells per 100-mm plate, one plate per student

16. After seeding the cells and adding sodium butyrate, image the cells. Transfer the plates to the incubator. Allow the cells to proliferate for one week. perform trypsinization and cell count on day 7.
17. Repeat the same setup as in step 15. Subculture cells from the control plate to a new control plate. Subculture cells from the sodium butyrate treatment to a new sodium butyrate treatment plate. Plate the suggested cell numbers in step 15 for each treatment. Allow the culture to proceed for 7 days. Repeat cell count on day 7.
18. Calculate the PDL using the formula in the Note box. From the data, calculate cumulative PDL and the number of hours for your cells to go through one round of replication (Table below).

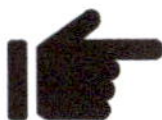

NOTE: PDL = 3.32 [log (total viable cells at harvest/total viable cells at seeding)]

19. Create a spreadsheet as shown Table IP 3.1. This allows you to keep track of the population doubling time more effectively. Plug in the formula for number of days, PDL and cPDL calculations and for average PDL time. You may also use the PDL spreadsheet template posted on the course site.

TABLE IP 3.1 Sample Data Sheet for PDL Study

Day of plating	Day of subculture	Days in culture	Cells seeded on day of plating	Today's yield	PDL	Cumulative PDL	Average PDL time (hours)
1/4/2018	1/7/2018	3	100,000	480,000	2.26	2.26	31.8
1/7/2018	1/13/2018	6	100,000	2,440,000	4.61	6.87	31.2
1/13/2018	1/19/2018	6	100,000	3,050,000	4.93	11.80	29.2
1/19/2018	1/25/2018	6	100,000	2,930,000	4.81	16.68	29.6
1/25/2018	1/31/2018	6	100,000	3,128,000	4.97	21.64	29.0
1/31/2018	2/6/2018	6	100,000	3,114,000	4.96	26.60	29.0

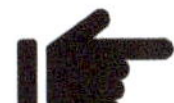

NOTE: If the yield of cells is too high or too low after 7 days in culture, you may adjust the seeding density for the specific treatment. However, make sure to note those changes in the spreadsheet.

Analysis

- Did you observe any difference in cell proliferation between the control plate and the sodium butyrate treatment?
- Are the differences statistically significant?
- Present your results graphically.
- Explain and discuss your results in your lab report. Base your discussion on published literature.

TROUBLESHOOTING: If large patches of cells still remain on the plate after step 3, perform the following steps:

a. Rinse the plate once *very gently* with DPBS(−).
b. Repeat trypsinization per regular protocol, with 3 ml of trypsin.
c. Check the plate under the microscope to monitor the degree of trypsinization.
d. After trypsinization, add 2 ml of complete medium for a total volume of 5 ml. Pipette vigorously to release the cells from the plate.
e. Collect 5 ml of cell suspension and pool this with the cell suspension already in the 15-ml tube from first isolation.

TABLE IP 3.2 Supply List: Vendors and Catalog Numbers

Item	Vendor	Catalog #
NIH/3T3 cells	ATCC	CRL-1658
Sodium butyrate 98%	VWR	103517-764
100 mm × 20 mm Tissue Culture Treated Dishes With Grip Ring	Chemglass	CLS-1805-152
DMEM media (with 4.5 g/L glucose and sodium pyruvate, without L-glutamine)	VWR	45000-316
Fetal bovine serum	Your choice	Multiple
Glutamax supplement (100x)	Thermo Fisher	35050061
Penicillin: streptomycin solution 100x, Corning	VWR	45000-652
DPBS(−)	VWR	45000-434
Four-Chip Disposable Hemocytometer, four chambers per chip	VWR	102966-632
Double Neubauer Chamber With Two Cover glasses	VWR	102094-780

Young Versus Old Primary Cells

Young Versus Old Mouse or Human Primary Cells

This is a more advanced independent team project. Students are provided with culture plates containing young (5–10 PDL) versus old cells (35 to 40 PDL). The challenge is for students to perform PDL study and determine which culture represents young cells and which culture represents old cells. Students will develop their own protocol to complete this project. Students will use their experience with the other PDL protocols (FBS concentration protocol, bFGF protocol, or sodium butyrate protocol) to plan and implement this study.

Reagents and Supplies

- Prepare your own complete media. Prepare 50 ml of complete media at a time in 50-ml tubes. Label them with your name or initials and date of media preparation. Save your tube in your assigned rack in the fridge. Prepare fresh complete media, as needed.

Procedure

1. Create your own protocol.
2. Determine the best cell density for cell seeding for once-a-week subculture.
3. If you decide to perform subculture frequently, discuss with your course instructor and justify the needs.
4. Feel free to consider the use of growth factors such as bFGF or EGF, if necessary. Again, discuss this with your course instructor to justify the use of growth factors.
   If using growth factors, determine the ideal concentrations for fibroblast culture.

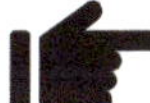

NOTE: PDL = 3.32 [log (total viable cells at harvest/total viable cells at seeding)]

5. Create a spreadsheet for each culture using the example provided in Table IP 4.1. The spreadsheet allows you to keep track of the population doubling time more effectively. Plug in the formula for number of days, PDL, and cPDL calculations as well as for average PDL time. You may also use the PDL spreadsheet template posted on the course site.

TABLE IP 4.1 Sample Data Sheet for PDL Study

Day of plating	Day of subculture	Days in culture	Cells seeded on day of plating	Today's yield	PDL	Cumulative PDL	Average PDL time (hours)
1/4/2018	1/7/2018	3	100,000	480,000	2.26	2.26	31.8
1/7/2018	1/13/2018	6	100,000	2,440,000	4.61	6.87	31.2
1/13/2018	1/19/2018	6	100,000	3,050,000	4.93	11.80	29.2
1/19/2018	1/25/2018	6	100,000	2,930,000	4.81	16.68	29.6
1/25/2018	1/31/2018	6	100,000	3,128,000	4.97	21.64	29.0
1/31/2018	2/6/2018	6	100,000	3,114,000	4.96	26.60	29.0

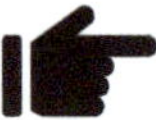

NOTE: If the yield of cells is too high or too low after 7 days in culture, you may adjust the seeding density for the specific treatment. However, make sure to note those changes in the spreadsheet.

Analysis

- Did you observe any difference in cell proliferation between the two cultures?
- Are you able to determine which primary cell line is young and which is getting closer to senescence?
- If one cell line has reached senescence, how would you definitively prove it?
- Are the differences statistically significant?
- Present your results graphically.
- Explain and discuss your results in your lab report. Base your discussion on published literature.

TROUBLESHOOTING: If large patches of cells still remain on the plate after step 3, perform the following steps:

a. Rinse the plate once *very gently* with DPBS(−).
b. Repeat trypsinization per regular protocol, with 3 ml of trypsin.
c. Check the plate under the microscope to monitor the degree of trypsinization.
d. After trypsinization, add 2 ml of complete medium for a total volume of 5 ml. Pipette vigorously to release the cells from the plate.

Collect 5 ml of cell suspension and pool this with the cell suspension already in the 15-ml tube from first isolation.

Surface Coating of Small PDMS Pieces, Cell Seeding, and Cell Growth

---

This independent team project is the culmination of all the procedures you have learned in the course thus far. Students are expected to do the following. Please understand that there is no detailed protocol for this procedure. Students are expected to write their own detailed procedure for this experiment and submit that along with the lab report:

1. Plan the project.
2. Choose the most suitable coating materials or combinations of coating materials based on the substrate coating protocol you did earlier in the term.
3. Plan to perform the study in stages or in one go. If you prefer the latter (one go), plan to be in the lab for about 7–8 hours (no kidding!). Plan to divide the labor between the team members based on each student's strengths and time availability.
4. Please set up a time to discuss the procedures with your course instructor before embarking on the project.
5. Make sure to discuss the experimental plan, incorporation of proper positive and negative controls, number of samples per treatment and *all* parameters you plan to employ in the project. This must include the following:

    a. coating materials
    b. preparation of coating material (including concentration of stock solutions, solvent used to prepare the coating materials, pH, temperature, etc.)
    c. sterilization techniques (for coating solutions and PDMS)
    d. type of culture vessels used for PDMS pieces
    e. number of replicates
    f. positive and negative controls
    g. duration of coating
    h. optimal cell droplet size to seed cells on small PDMS pieces
    i. optimal cell density and total cell number per PDMS piece (see serial dilution or equivalent methods)
    j. optimum time for cell attachment

k. ways to prevent droplet evaporation during the time of cell attachment (can be up to 2 to 4 hours)
l. Determine the best adhesive to keep the PDMS pieces attached to the well for 7 days immersed in culture medium. The glue should be biocompatible and non toxic (see materials used in the **Biocompatability and toxicity testing** experiment on page 145). The glue should be transparent enough to obtain undistorted images.
m. precautions while flooding the wells with complete media
n. imaging, soon after seeding the droplets, right before and after flooding
o. the time points for further imaging (days 3, 5, and 7, as applicable)

This project, therefore, encompasses the following procedures:

- subculturing of cells
- cell counting
- contact angle measurement
- surface coating treatments
- biocompatibility/toxicity testing
- serial dilution of cells and seeding specific cell numbers on a 1" × 1" piece of PDMS
- most importantly, planning an experiment, estimating the time to complete the seeding procedure, and imaging cells on top of PDMS pieces

Please refer to the protocols in the Preparation for Independent Projects section to prepare for this project. Refer to your lab notebook for specifics.

APPENDICES

Appendix I

Biosafety Levels Infographic

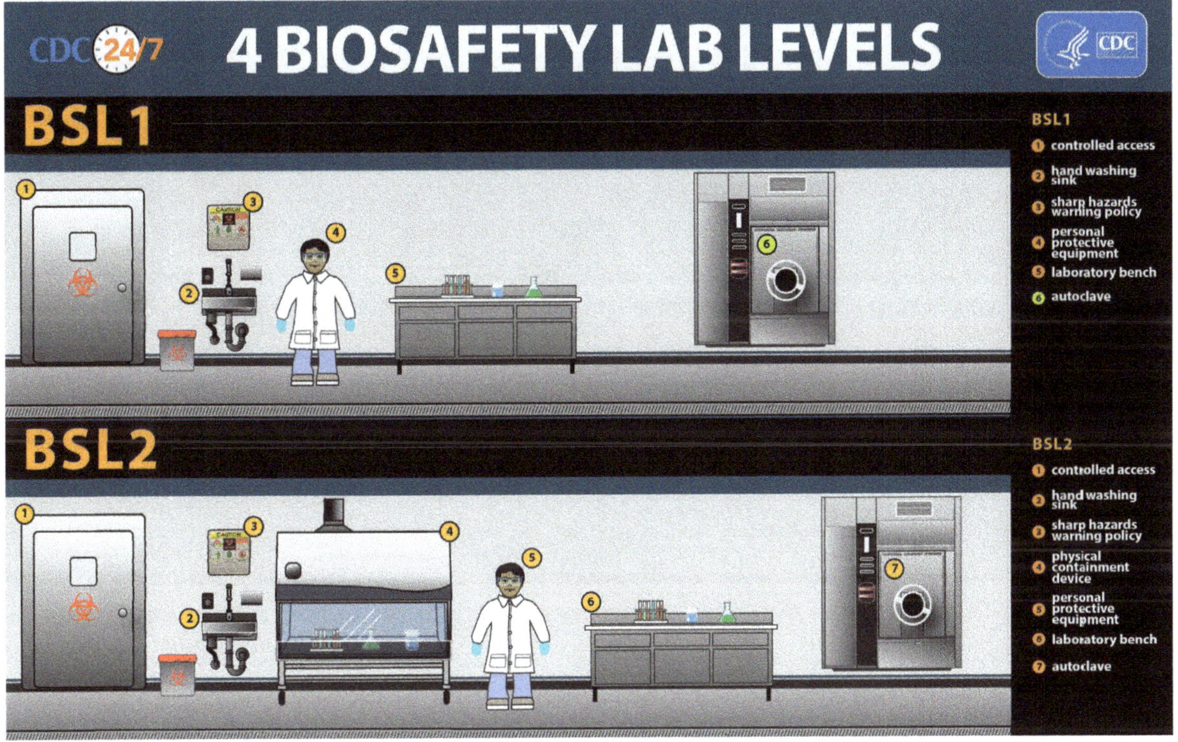

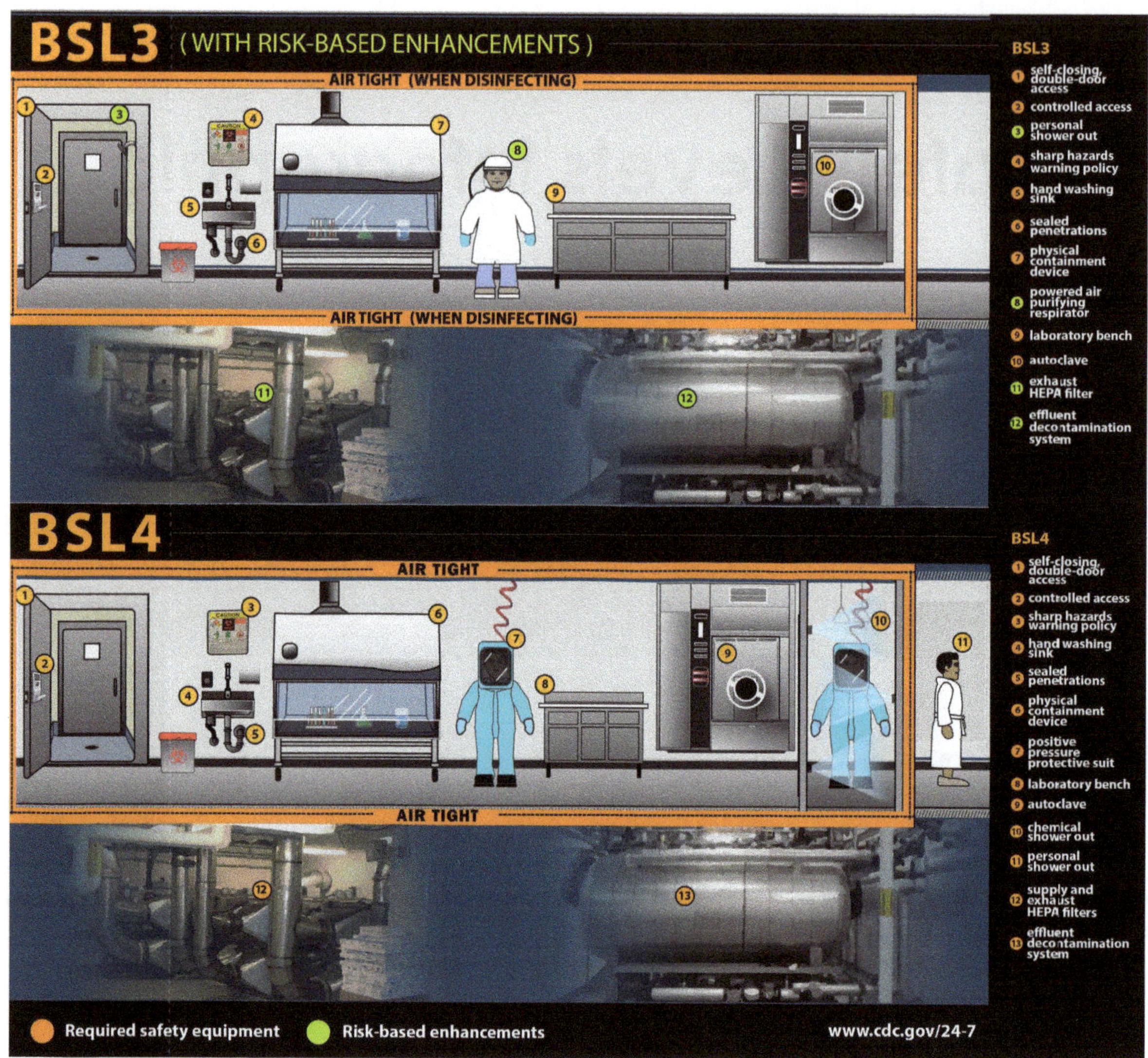

FIGURE A1 CDC, "Biosafety Levels," https://www.cdc.gov/orr/infographics/biosafety.htm.

Appendix II

Biosafety Levels

Biosafety Level 1 (BSL-1)

BSL-1 labs are used to study infectious agents or toxins not known to consistently cause disease in healthy adults. They follow basic safety procedures, called Standard Microbiological Practices, and require no special equipment or design features. Standard engineering controls in BSL-1 laboratories include easily cleaned surfaces that are able to withstand the basic chemicals used in the laboratory. Some examples of BSL-1 organisms include *Agrobacterium radiobacter*, *Aspergillus niger*, *Bacillus thuringiensis*, *Escherichia coli strain K12*, *Lactobacillus acidophilus*, *Micrococcus leuteus*, *Neurospora crassa*, *Pseudomonas fluorescens*, and *Serratia marcescens*.

Biosafety Level 2 (BSL-2)

BSL-2 laboratories are used to study moderate-risk infectious agents or toxins that pose a risk if accidentally inhaled, swallowed, or exposed to the skin. Examples of BSL-2 organisms include equine encephalitis viruses, HIV, lentivirus, mycobacterium, *Streptococcus pneumonia*, and *Salmonella choleraesuis*. Design requirements for BSL-2 laboratories include handwashing sinks, eyewash stations, and doors that close automatically and lock. BSL-2 labs must also have access to equipment that can decontaminate laboratory waste, including an incinerator, an autoclave, and/or another method, depending on the biological risk assessment.

Biosafety Level 3 (BSL-3)

BSL-3 laboratories are used to study infectious agents or toxins that may be transmitted through the air and cause potentially lethal infection through inhalation exposure. Researchers perform all experiments in biosafety cabinets that use carefully controlled air flow or sealed enclosures to prevent infection. BSL-3 laboratories are designed to be easily decontaminated. These laboratories must use

U.S. Department of Health and Human Services, Selection from "Biosafety Levels," *Science Safety Security*, U.S. Department of Health and Human Services, 2015.

controlled, or "directional," air flow to ensure air flows from nonlaboratory areas (such as the hallway) into laboratory areas as an additional safety measure. BSL-3 examples include yellow fever, West Nile virus, and *Mycobacterium tuberculosis*.

Other engineered safety features include the use of two self-closing, or interlocked, doors; sealed windows and wall surfaces; and filtered ventilation systems. BSL-3 labs must also have access to equipment that can decontaminate laboratory waste, including an incinerator, an autoclave, and/or another method, depending on the biological risk assessment.

Biosafety Level 4 (BSL-4)

BSL-4 laboratories are used to study infectious agents or toxins that pose a high risk of aerosol-transmitted laboratory infections and life-threatening disease for which no vaccine or therapy is available. Examples include Ebola, Marburg viruses, Lassa fever, Bolivian hemorrhagic fever, and many other hemorrhagic viruses found in the tropics. The laboratories incorporate all BSL 3 features and occupy safe, isolated zones within a larger building or may be housed in a separate, dedicated building. Access to BSL-4 laboratories is carefully controlled and requires significant training.

There are two types of BSL-4 laboratories:

cabinet laboratory: all work with infectious agents or toxins is done in a class III biosafety cabinet with very carefully designed procedures to contain any potential contamination. In addition, the laboratory space is designed to also prevent contamination of other spaces.

suit laboratory: Laboratory personnel are required to wear full-body, air-supplied suits, which are the most sophisticated type of personal protective equipment. All personnel shower before exiting the laboratory and go through a series of procedures designed to fully decontaminate them before leaving.

The engineering controls required are different for BSL-4 cabinet and suit laboratories. For either type, they are extensive and supplemented by carefully designed procedures and practices. For more information about the biosafety level guidelines, refer to *Biosafety in Microbiological and Biomedical Laboratories, 5th Edition,* which is available at www.cdc.gov/od/ohs/biosfty/bmbl5/bmbl5toc.htm.

Reference

Centers for Disease Control and Prevention. (2020). *Biosafety in microbiological and biomedical laboratories* (6th ed.). https://www.cdc.gov/labs/BMBL.html

Appendix III

Buffer Composition

Composition of 1X Phosphate Buffered Saline

Components	Mole. Weight (g/mol)	Grams/Liter (g)	Molarity (mM)
Sodium Chloride (NaCl)	58.44	8.0	136.9
Potassium Chloride (KCl)	74.55	0.2	2.67
Sodium Phosphate Dibasic (Na_2HPO_4)	141.96	1.42	10
Potassium Phosphate Monobasic (KH_2PO_4)	136.09	0.24	1.8

Composition of 1X Dulbecco's Phosphate Buffered Saline Without Calcium and Magnesium (DPBS−)

Components	Mole. Weight (g/mol)	Grams/Liter (g)	Molarity (mM)
Potassium Chloride (KCl)	74.55	0.2	2.67
Sodium Chloride (NaCl)	58.44	8.0	136.9
Potassium Phosphate Monobasic (KH_2PO_4)	136.09	0.2	1.47
Sodium Phosphate Dibasic, anhydrous (Na_2HPO_4)	141.96	1.15	8.10
pH to 7.2–7.4			

Composition of 1X Dulbecco's Phosphate Buffered Saline With Calcium and Magnesium (DPBS+)

Components	Mole. Weight (g/mol)	Grams/Liter (g)	Molarity (mM)
Potassium Chloride (KCl)	74.55	0.2	2.67
Sodium Chloride (NaCl)	58.44	8.0	136.9
Potassium Phosphate Monobasic (KH_2PO_4)	136.09	0.2	1.47
Sodium Phosphate Dibasic (Na_2HPO_4)	141.96	1.15	8.10
Calcium Chloride ($CaCl_2$)	110.98	0.1	0.90
Magnesium Chloride ($MgCl_2 \cdot 6H_20$)	203.30	0.1	0.50

Procedure to Prepare PBS, DPBS (–), and DPBS (+)

Add 800 ml distilled water to a 1 L measuring cylinder. While stirring with a magnetic stirrer bar, add the individual components in sequence and stir until the salts are completely dissolved in water. Adjust the pH to the desired pH using 1N HCL or 1N NaOH, typically 7.4 for cell culture procedures. Once the pH is stabilized, add distilled water to bring the final volume to 1 L. Sterilize the solution either by autoclaving or filtering through a 0.22 micron filter.

Composition of 1X Hank's Balanced Salt Solution (HBSS) With Calcium and Magnesium

Components	Mole. Weight (g/mol)	Grams/Liter (g)	Molarity (mM)
Sodium Chloride (NaCl)	58.44	8.0	137
Potassium Chloride (KCl)	74.55	0.4	5.37
Calcium Chloride ($CaCl_2$)	110.98	0.14	1.26
Magnesium Sulfate Heptahydrate ($MgSO_4 \cdot 7H_2O$)	246.47	0.1	0.41
Magnesium Chloride Hexahydrate ($MgCl_2 \cdot 6H2O$)	203.30	0.1	0.49
Sodium Phosphate Dibasic Dihydrate ($Na_2HPO_4 \cdot 2H_2O$)	177.99	0.048*	0.27
Potassium Phosphate Monobasic (KH_2PO_4)	136.09	0.06	0.44
Sodium bicarbonate ($NaHCO_3$)	84.01	0.35	4.17
D-Glucose (Dextrose)	180.16	1.0	5.55

Composition of 1X Hank's Balanced Salt Solution (HBSS) Without Calcium and Magnesium

Components	Mole. Weight (g/mol)	Grams/Liter (g)	Molarity (mM)
Sodium Chloride (NaCl)	58.44	8.0	137
Potassium Chloride (KCl)	74.55	0.4	5.37
Sodium Phosphate Dibasic Dihydrate ($Na_2HPO_4 \cdot 2H_2O$)	177.99	0.048*	0.27
Potassium Phosphate Monobasic (KH_2PO_4)	136.09	0.06	0.44
Sodium bicarbonate ($NaHCO_3$)	84.01	0.35	4.17
D-Glucose (Dextrose)	180.16	1.0	5.55

*some recipes indicate suggest 0.06 g of Na_2HPO_4 (0.34 mM)

Procedure to Prepare HBSS

Add 800 ml distilled water to a 1 L measuring cylinder. While stirring with a magnetic stirrer bar, add the individual components in sequence and stir until the components are completely dissolved in water. Adjust the pH to the desired pH using 1N HCL or 1N NaOH, typically 7.4 for cell culture procedures. Once the pH is stabilized, add distilled water to bring the final volume to 1 L. Sterilize the solution by filtering through a 0.22 micron filter. Applications where addition of phenol red is indicated, add phenol red (powder or a high concentration stock solution) to 33 μM final concentration. If using phenol red stock solution, add it before making up the final 1 L volume.

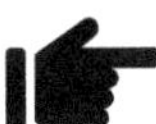

NOTE: Solutions containing glucose should only be filter sterilized to prevent charring when glucose is autoclaved.

Since HBSS contains glucose, it should be sterilized only by filtration.

Appendix IV

DMEM Medium Formulations

CORNING

DMEM

Formulation

Cat. No.	10-013	10-014	10-017	10-027	10-101	10-102	15-013	15-017	15-018
Description	Liquid, 1x	Liquid, 1x	Liquid, 1x	Liquid, 1x	Liquid, 1x	Liquid, 1x	Liquid, 1x	Liquid, 1x	Liquid, 1x
Units	mg/L	mg/L	mg/L	mg/L	mg/L	mg/L	mg/L	mg/L	mg/L
Components									
Inorganic Salts									
$CaCl_2$ (anhydrous)	200	200	200	200	200	200	200	200	200
$Fe(NO_3)_3 \cdot 9H_2O$	0.1	0.1	0.1	0.1	0.1	0.1	0.1	0.1	0.1
KCl	400	400	400	400	400	400	400	400	400
$MgSO_4$ (anhydrous)	97.7	97.7	97.7	97.7	97.7	97.7	97.7	97.7	97.7
NaCl	6400	6400	6400	4750	6400	6400	6400	6400	6400
$NaH2PO_4 \cdot H_2O$	125	125	125	125	125	125	125	125	125
$NaHCO_3$	3700	3700	3700	3700	3700	3700	3700	3700	3700
Amino Acids									
L-Arginine • HCl	84	84	84	84	84	84	84	84	84.00
L-Cystine • 2HCl	62.57	62.57	62.57	62.57	62.57	62.57	62.57	62.57	62.57
L-Alanyi-L-glutamine	—	—	—	—	869	869	—	—	—
L-Glutamine	584	584	584	584	—	—	—	—	—
Glycine	30	30	30	30	30	30	30	30	30.00
L-Histidine •HCl • H_2O	42	42	42	42	42	42	42	42	42.00
L-Isoleucine	104.8	104.8	104.8	104.8	104.8	104.8	104.8	104.8	104.80
L-Leucine	104.8	104.8	104.8	104.8	104.8	104.8	104.8	104.8	104.80
L-Lysine • HCl	146.2	146.2	146.2	146.2	146.2	146.2	146.2	146.2	146.20
L-Methionine	30	30	30	30	30	30	30	30	30.00
L-Phenylalanine	66	66	66	66	66	66	66	66	66.00
L-Serine	42	42	42	42	42	42	42	42	42.00
L-Threonine	95.2	95.2	95.2	95.2	95.2	95.2	95.2	95.2	95.20
L-Tryptophan	16	16	16	16	16	16	16	16	16.00
L-Tyrosine • 2Na • $2H_2O$	103.79	103.79	103.79	103.79	103.79	103.79	103.79	103.79	103.79
L-Valine	94	94	94	94	94	94	94	94	94.00

Vitamins									
D-Calcium pantothenate	4.00	4.00	4.00	4.00	4.00	4.00	4.00	4.00	4.00
Choline chloride	4.00	4.00	4.00	4.00	4.00	4.00	4.00	4.00	4.00
Folic acid	4.00	4.00	4.00	4.00	4.00	4.00	4.00	4.00	4.00
i-Inositol	7.20	7.20	7.20	7.20	7.20	7.20	7.20	7.20	7.20
Nicotinamide	4.00	4.00	4.00	4.00	4.00	4.00	4.00	4.00	4.00
Pyridoxine • HCl	4.00	4.00	4.00	4.00	4.00	4.00	4.00	4.00	4.00
Riboflavin	0.40	0.40	0.40	0.40	0.40	0.40	0.40	0.40	0.40
Thiamine • HCl	4.00	4.00	4.00	4.00	4.00	4.00	4.00	4.00	4.00
Other									
D-Glucose	4500.00	1000.00	4500.00	4500.00	4500.00	4500.00	4500.00	4500.00	4500.00
Phenol red • Na	15.00	15.00	15.00	15.00	15.00	15.00	15.00	15.00	15.00
Sodium pyruvate	110.00	110.00	—	—	110.00	—	110.00	—	110.00
HEPES	—	—	—	5958.00	—	—	—	—	5958.00

Add									
L-Glutamine									
Powder (mg/L)	—	—	—	—	—	—	584.00	584.00	584.00
200 mM Solution (mL/L)	—	—	—	—	—	—	20.00	20.00	20.00

Cat. No.	**17-204**	**17-205**	**17-207**	**50-003**	**50-013**	**90-013**	**90-113**
Description	**Liquid, 1x**	**Liquid, 1x**	**Liquid, 1x**	**Powder**	**Powder**	**Powder**	**Powder**
Units	**mg/L**	**mg/L**	**mg/L**	**mg/L**	**mg/L**	**mg/L**	**mg/L**
Components							
Inorganic Salts							
$CaCl_2$ (anhydrous)	200	200.00	200.00	200.00	200.00	200.00	200.00
$Fe(NO_3)_3 \cdot 9H_2O$	0.1	0.10	0.10	0.10	0.10	0.10	0.10
KCl	400	400.00	400.00	400.00	400.00	400.00	400.00
$MgSO_4$ (anhydrous)	97.7	97.70	97.70	97.70	97.70	97.70	97.70
NaCl	6400	6400.00	6400.00	6400.00	6400.00	6400.00	6400.00
$NaH_2PO_4 \cdot H_2O$	125	125.00	125.00	125.00	125.00	125.00	125.00
$NaHCO_3$	3700	3700.00	3700.00	—	—	—	—
Amino Acids							
L-Arginine • HCl	84.00	84.00	84.00	84.00	84.00	84.00	84.00
L-Cystine • 2HCl	—	62.57	62.57	62.57	62.57	62.57	62.57
L-Glutamine	—	—	—	584.00	584.00	—	—
Glycine	30.00	30.00	30.00	30.00	30.00	30.00	30.00
L-Histidine • HCl • H_2O	42.00	42.00	42.00	42.00	42.00	42.00	42.00
L-Isoleucine	104.80	104.80	104.80	104.80	104.80	104.80	104.80
L-Leucine	104.80	104.80	104.80	104.80	104.80	104.80	104.80
L-Lysine • HCl	146.20	146.20	146.20	146.20	146.20	146.20	146.20
L-Methionine	—	30.00	30.00	30.00	30.00	30.00	30.00
L-Phenylalanine	66.00	66.00	66.00	66.00	66.00	66.00	66.00
L-Serine	42.00	42.00	42.00	42.00	42.00	42.00	42.00
L-Threonine	95.20	95.20	95.20	95.20	95.20	95.20	95.20
L-Tryptophan	16.00	16.00	16.00	16.00	16.00	16.00	16.00
L-Tyrosine • 2Na • $2H_2O$	103.79	103.79	103.79	103.79	103.79	103.79	103.79
L-Valine	94.00	94.00	94.00	94.00	94.00	94.00	94.00

Cat. No.	17-204	17-205	17-207	50-003	50-013	90-013	90-113
Description	**Liquid, 1x**	**Liquid, 1x**	**Liquid, 1x**	**Powder**	**Powder**	**Powder**	**Powder**
Units	**mg/L**	**mg/L**	**mg/L**	**mg/L**	**mg/L**	**mg/L**	**mg/L**
Components							
Inorganic Salts							
$CaCl_2$ (anhydrous)	200	200.00	200.00	200.00	200.00	200.00	200.00
$Fe(NO_3)_3 \cdot 9H_2O$	0.1	0.10	0.10	0.10	0.10	0.10	0.10
KCl	400	400.00	400.00	400.00	400.00	400.00	400.00
$MgSO_4$ (anhydrous)	97.7	97.70	97.70	97.70	97.70	97.70	97.70
NaCl	6400	6400.00	6400.00	6400.00	6400.00	6400.00	6400.00
$NaH_2PO_4 \cdot H_2O$	125	125.00	125.00	125.00	125.00	125.00	125.00
$NaHCO_3$	3700	3700.00	3700.00	—	—	—	—
Amino Acids							
L-Arginine • HCl	84.00	84.00	84.00	84.00	84.00	84.00	84.00
L-Cystine • 2HCl	—	62.57	62.57	62.57	62.57	62.57	62.57
L-Glutamine	—	—	—	584.00	584.00	—	—
Glycine	30.00	30.00	30.00	30.00	30.00	30.00	30.00
L-Histidine •HCl • H_2O	42.00	42.00	42.00	42.00	42.00	42.00	42.00
L-Isoleucine	104.80	104.80	104.80	104.80	104.80	104.80	104.80
L-Leucine	104.80	104.80	104.80	104.80	104.80	104.80	104.80
L-Lysine • HCl	146.20	146.20	146.20	146.20	146.20	146.20	146.20
L-Methionine	—	30.00	30.00	30.00	30.00	30.00	30.00
L-Phenylalanine	66.00	66.00	66.00	66.00	66.00	66.00	66.00
L-Serine	42.00	42.00	42.00	42.00	42.00	42.00	42.00
L-Threonine	95.20	95.20	95.20	95.20	95.20	95.20	95.20
L-Tryptophan	16.00	16.00	16.00	16.00	16.00	16.00	16.00
L-Tyrosine • 2Na • $2H_2O$	103.79	103.79	103.79	103.79	103.79	103.79	103.79
L-Valine	94.00	94.00	94.00	94.00	94.00	94.00	94.00
Vitamins							
D-Calcium pantothenate	4.00	4.00	4.00	4.00	4.00	4.00	4.00
Choline chloride	4.00	4.00	4.00	4.00	4.00	4.00	4.00
Folic acid	4.00	4.00	4.00	4.00	4.00	4.00	4.00
i-Inositol	7.20	7.20	7.20	7.20	7.20	7.20	7.20
Nicotinamide	4.00	4.00	4.00	4.00	4.00	4.00	4.00
Pyridoxine • HCl	4.00	4.00	4.00	4.00	4.00	4.00	4.00
Riboflavin	0.40	0.40	0.40	0.40	0.40	0.40	0.40
Thiamine • HCl	4.00	4.00	4.00	4.00	4.00	4.00	4.00
Other							
D-Glucose	4500.00	4500.00	—	4500.00	4500.00	4500.00	—
Phenol red • Na	15.00	—	15.00	15.00	15.00	—	—
Sodium pyruvate	110.00	110.00	—	110.00	—	—	—
HEPES	—	—	—	—	—	—	—
Add							
$NaHCO_3$ Powder (g/L) 7.5% Solution (mL/L)	 — —	 — —	 — —	 3.70 49.40	 3.70 49.40	 — —	 3.70 49.40
L-Glutamine Powder (mg/L) 200 mM Solution (mL/L)	 584.00 20.00	 584.00 20.00	 584.00 20.00	 — —	 — —	 — —	 584.00 20.00

Appendix V

Surface Areas and Guide for Recommended Medium Volumes

Corning® Microplates

Microplate	Well Diameter (Bottom) (mm)	Single Well Only: Approx. Growth Area (cm^2)	Average Cell Yield	Total Well Volume (µL)	Working Volume (µL)
Corning 96-well Microplates					
Flat Bottom	6.4	0.32	3.2×10^4	360	100 – 200
Round Bottom	6.4	N/A**	N/A**	330	100 – 200
V-Bottom	6.4	0.38	3.8×10^4	320	100 – 200
Half Area	4.5	0.16	1.6×10^4	190	50 – 100
Corning 384-well Microplates					
Standard	2.7 x 2.7*	0.056	5.6×10^3	112	25 – 50
Low Volume	2.0	0.031	3.1×10^3	50	5 – 40
Corning 1536-well Microplates					
Low Volume	1.2	0.011	1.2×10^3	2.3	1 – 1.5
Clear Flat Bottom	1.63*	0.025	2.5×10^3	12.5	5 – 10
Solid Flat Bottom	1.53*	0.023	2.3×10^3	12.5	5 – 10

*Square wells.
**Because these wells are round, the surface area available for cell attachment is dependent on the medium volume used.

Corning Multiple Well Plates

Plate	Well Diameter (Bottom) (mm)	Single Well Only: Approx. Growth Area (cm²)	Average Cell Yield	Total Well Volume (mL)	Working Volume (mL)
6-well	34.8	9.5	9.5×10^5	16.8	1.9 – 2.9
12-well	22.1	3.8	3.8×10^5	6.9	0.76 – 1.14
24-well	15.6	1.9	1.9×10^5	3.4	0.38 – 0.57
48-well	11.0	0.95	9.5×10^4	1.6	0.19 – 0.285

Transwell® Permeable Supports

Transwell Insert Format	Transwell Insert Diameter (mm)	Approx. Growth Area (cm²)	Average Cell Yield	Recommended Volume (mL)	
				Well	Insert
6-well	24 mm	4.67 cm²	4.67×10^5	2.6	1.5
12-well	12 mm	1.12 cm²	1.12×10^5	1.5	0.5
24-well	6.5 mm	0.33 cm²	3.3×10^4	0.6	0.1
96-well	4.26 mm	0.143 cm²	1.4×10^4	0.235	0.075
100 mm dish	75 mm	44 cm²	4.4×10^6	13.0	9.0

Corning Dishes

Dish	Approx. Growth Area (cm²)	Average Cell Yield	Recommended Volume (mL)
35 mm*	9	9.0×10^5	1.8 – 2.7
60 mm*	21	2.1×10^6	4.2 – 6.3
100 mm*	55	5.5×10^6	11 – 16.5
150 mm*	152	1.52×10^7	30.4 – 45.6
245 mm†	500	5.0×10^7	100 – 150

*Not actual bottom diameters.
†Dish is square.

Corning® Flasks***

Flask	Approx. Growth Area (cm²)	Average Cell Yield	Recommended Medium Volume (mL)	Approx. Total Flask Volume (mL)
25 cm²	25	2.5×10^6	5 – 7.5	70 rectangular
75 cm²	75	7.5×10^6	15 – 22.5	265 U-shaped
150 cm²	150	1.5×10^7	30 – 45	377 U-shaped
175 cm²	175	1.75×10^7	35 – 52.5	513 U-shaped
225 cm²	225	2.25×10^7	45 – 67.5	1,006 traditional
Corning HYPER*Flask*®	1,720	1.72×10^8	560 – 565	560 – 565

***Corning flasks (larger than 100 cm²) are considered US Class I medical devices.

Corning Stacked Chambers***

Chamber Size	Approximate Growth Area (cm²)	Average Cell Yield	Recommended Medium Volume (mL)
Corning CellSTACK® Chambers			
1-stack	636	6.36×10^7	127–191
2-stack	1,272	1.27×10^8	254–382
5-stack	3,180	3.18×10^8	636–954
10-stack	6,360	6.36×10^8	1,272–1,908
40-stack	25,440	2.54×10^9	5,088–7,632
Corning HYPER*Stack*® Chambers			
12-stack	6,000	6.0×10^8	1,300
36-stack	18,000	1.8×10^9	3,900

***Corning stacked chambers are considered US Class I medical devices.

Corning Roller Bottles***

Roller Bottle	Approximate Growth Area (cm²)	Average Cell Yield	Recommended Medium Volume (mL)
490 cm²	490	4.9×10^7	100–150
850 cm²	850	8.5×10^7	170–255
1,700 cm² ESRB	1,700	1.7×10^8	340–510
1,750 cm²	1,750	1.75×10^8	350–525

***Corning roller bottles are considered US Class I medical devices.

Corning CellCube® Systems***

CellCube Module	Approximate Growth Area (cm²)	Average Cell Yield	Recommended Medium Volume (mL)
10-stack	8,500	8.5×10^8	N/A*
25-stack	21,250	2.13×10^9	N/A*
50-stack	42,500	4.25×10^9	N/A*
100-stack	85,000	8.5×10^9	N/A*

*Not applicable; these systems are perfused with medium from a reservoir.
***Corning CellCube systems are considered US Class I medical devices.

Appendix VI

Definitions of Terms Frequently Used in Tissue Culture

anchorage dependence: the requirement for attachment for cells to proliferate

anchorage independence: the ability of cells to proliferate in suspension, either stirred or suspended in agar or Methocel

authentication: corroboration of the identity of a cell line with reference to its origin

cell concentration: the number of cells per ml of medium

cell density: the number of cells per cm^2 of growth surface

cell line: the progeny of a primary culture when it is subcultured; a cell line may be **finite** or **continuous**

cell strains: cell lines that have been purified by physical separation, selection, or cloning and which have specific defined characteristics; for example, BHK-21-PyY, anchorage-independent cells cloned from the BHK-21 cell line following transformation with polyoma virus

cloning or cell cloning: the generation of a colony from a single cell, and subculture of such a colony would give rise to a cell strain; because of potential confusion with molecular cloning, this term is probably better modified as "cell cloning"

confluence: a cell density at which all cells are in contact with no remaining growth surface

contact inhibition: strictly, the loss of plasma membrane ruffling and cell motility on contact in confluent cultures but often used to imply loss of cell proliferation after confluence—better referred to as **density limitation of cell proliferation**

continuous cell line: a cell line with an indefinite lifespan (immortal, over 100 population doublings; see also **immortalization**)

density limitation of cell proliferation: the reduction or cessation of cell proliferation at high cell density

differentiation: acquisition of properties characteristic of the fully functional cell in vivo

DNA profiling: the assay of hypervariable regions of satellite DNA, usually by determining the frequency of short tandem repeats in microsatellite DNA, using PCR of individual loci with defined primers

established cell line: the use of this term is discouraged because it is ambiguous; the preferred term is **continuous cell line**

explantation: isolation of tissue for maintenance in vitro

finite cell line: a cell line that survives for a fixed number of population doublings—usually 40–60, before senescing and ceasing proliferation

generation number: the number of population doublings of a cell line since isolation

growth curve: a plot of cell number on a log scale against time on a linear scale

immortalization: the indefinite extension of lifespan in culture, usually achieved by genetic modification, but already acquired by some cancer cells

passage: the event of **subculture**, used to define the number of subcultures that a cell line has gone through since isolation; if used of **continuous cell lines**, usually the number of subcultures since last thawed from storage

primary culture: a culture from the time of isolation until its first subculture

primary explant: a small cellular fragment removed from tissue and placed in culture

provenance: details of the origin and life history of a cell line, including various accidental and deliberate manipulations that may have a significant effect on its properties, latent or expressed

split ratio: the amount by which a culture is diluted before reseeding—usually, a whole number

subculture: the transfer of cells from one culture vessel to another by dissociation from the substrate, if a monolayer, or by dilution, if grown in suspension

transformation: a heritable change involving an alteration in the genotype, usually subsequent to immortalization—best reserved for describing an alteration in growth characteristics associated with malignancy (**anchorage independence**, loss of **contact inhibition**, **density limitation of cell proliferation**, and **tumorigenesis in vivo**)

tumorigenesis: formation of a tumor in vivo—in the current context, from implanted cells or tissue

Reference

Geraghty, R. J., Capes-Davis, A., Davis J. M,, Downward, J., Freshney, R. I., Knezevic, I., Lovell-Badge, R., Masters, J. R., Meredith, J., Stacey, G. N., Thraves, P., Vias, M., & Cancer Research UK. (2014). Guidelines for the use of cell lines in biomedical research. *British Journal of Cancer*, *111*(6), 1021–46. https://www.doi.org/10.1038/bjc.2014.166. PMID: 25117809; PMCID: PMC4453835.